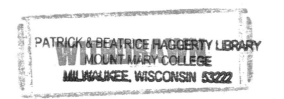
Real Solutions Weight Loss Workbook

Toni Piechota, MS, RD

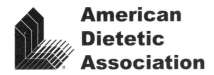

American Dietetic Association

Diana Faulhaber, Publisher
Laura Brown, Development Editor
Elizabeth Nishiura, Production Editor

The views expressed in this publication are those of the authors and do not necessarily reflect policies and/or official positions of the American Dietetic Association. Mention of product names in this publication does not constitute endorsement by the authors or the American Dietetic Association. The American Dietetic Association disclaims responsibility for the application of the information contained herein.

10 9 8 7 6 5 4 3 2 1

Library of Congress Cataloging-in-Publication Data

Piechota, Toni.
  Real solutions weight loss workbook / by Toni Piechota.
      p. cm.
  ISBN 0-88091-323-1
  1. Weight loss--Psychological aspects. 2. Behavior modification. I.
Title.

  RM222.2.P497 2003
  613.7'12--dc22

                                  2003014672

Contents

Preface

Real Solutions Weight Loss Workbook provides practical guidance for people seeking to lose weight and maintain weight loss and for health professionals working in the weight-loss field. This engaging workbook incorporates the principles of behavior modification: self-monitoring, realistic goal setting, and creating an environment that does not promote overeating. Negative self-talk and low self-efficacy interfere with effective weight control. *Real Solutions Weight Loss Workbook* guides the reader by challenging these negative thoughts through cognitive restructuring and thought-changing exercises. This workbook includes meal patterns, calorie tables, food record forms, and sample contracts for reference. The workbook presents basic facts about weight loss, safe and effective activity guidelines, and information on calculating and evaluating body mass index in an easy-to-understand format. *Real Solutions Weight Loss Workbook* is a comprehensive tool that both informs and encourages thought and action by the reader.

Introduction

In the early 1990s, the National Health and Nutrition Examination Survey (NHANES), conducted by the National Center for Health Statistics (NCHS), revealed that more than one in two adult Americans was overweight (defined as a body mass index of 25 or above), and almost one in four was obese (defined as a body mass index of 30 or above). Nationwide efforts were made to promote physical activity and low-fat, healthy diets. The public was made aware of the health risks of obesity. The food industry developed fat-free ice cream, cookies, cheese, and hot dogs. Even fast-food restaurants became healthier, with grilled chicken salads, sandwiches, and "lite burritos." The U.S. surgeon general determined that one of the primary health objectives of the country would be to reduce the incidence of obesity. According to NHANES studies from 1999 to 2000, however, *64 percent of Americans were now overweight, and 30 percent obese!* What happened?

Beginning Self-exploration

Part of the problem is the fact that efforts to reduce obesity have centered mostly around *education*. Of course, the first step in changing is becoming informed. But having information is only part of the solution. Many obese individuals have made several prior attempts at weight loss and know more about the subject than the "experts" do. It has been said before: *Knowledge does not equal behavior.* Eating has many roles in people's lives; and if individuals are to avoid using food to meet those needs, they must find other ways of getting them met. This is where self-exploration comes in. By becoming aware of how food serves you and what your specific areas of concern are, you place yourself in a position to find solutions.

Further, the decision to lose weight must be the decision to adopt a lifetime of new choices and behaviors. Some studies state that as many as 95 percent of people who lose weight gain it back. Many people try the "quick-fix" approach to weight loss—eating "wonder foods" that burn more calories than they contain and taking "wonder drugs" that are "scientifically proven" to "increase metabolic rate." Then there are the "wonder diets" guaranteed to help you lose 10 pounds in 10 days. Eat all the food you want! (Just make sure you get in your 20 ounces of mashed zucchini before each meal.) Of course, such claims are not valid. People who fall for these weight-loss programs generally don't lose weight.

Dieting and physical activity require a huge commitment, lots of support, adequate knowledge, and plenty of energy (both emotional and physical). Some people don't realize what is involved in losing weight and maintaining weight loss. When the going gets tough, these people choose a new goal. You must realize what you are committing to in initiating and maintaining weight loss, both to avoid surprises and to allow you to set appropriate goals for your motivation level.

Facing the Challenge

Losing and maintaining weight may be the biggest challenge you've ever faced in your life. This workbook is based on sound principles of nutrition and physical activity combined with a cognitive-behavioral approach to weight loss. What exactly does that mean? *Cognitive* means "thinking" or "having to do with thoughts." The cognitive part of the program addresses the way you think of yourself, weight, weight loss, and your ability to lose weight. Psychologists have found that these factors have a large impact on the way we act. And of course, weight is the result of many actions. Addressing the way you think about yourself and weight loss is the foundation for starting a weight-loss program.

Behavioral refers to actions, and *behavior modification* is a science that involves the use of specific strategies to replace undesirable behaviors with desirable behaviors. Part of this behavior modification program will include identifying your current behaviors, identifying factors that trigger those behaviors, and establishing systems of reward to reinforce desirable behaviors. By addressing such issues, you will find that the basic principles of weight loss that have been useless to you so far will have much more meaning.

"I Do . . ."
—Dieting and Commitment

Permanent weight loss can be the most difficult challenge a person ever faces. As in a marriage, a serious commitment is essential in weight loss. Throughout the process, there will undoubtedly be many obstacles. Part of ensuring long-term success is having a strong commitment and being prepared to deal with the inevitable difficulties you will face.

The Stages of Commitment

Prior to making a firm commitment to a major decision, most people go through several stages. Rarely do individuals wake up, decide that they are unhappy with some aspect of their lives, and at that moment make permanent changes to amend the situation. For most people, even the decision as to whether or not there exists a problem involves time and contemplation. They start to think that things are not right. They ask themselves certain questions: Is it me? Is it the environment? Did I not get enough sleep? Do I need more coffee? They may wonder if this dissatisfaction is something to worry about, or whether this "problem" will just blow over. After they accept that there is a problem, they contemplate the idea that maybe they should take some action. Perhaps they clearly feel that there is a problem that needs to be addressed, but they aren't sure how they can change it. Or maybe they know the solution but are not sure they are ready to face it. They may experience *denial* and think, "Well, maybe it's not that bad." In this way they avoid the issue. Some people spend a lot of time in this stage.

Something may happen, though, that jars an individual out of this stage. It may be something sudden. For example, people speak of very specific events that served as turning points for them. One woman sat in a chair at a party, and when the chair broke from underneath her, she was so overwhelmed with embarrassment that she realized that her weight was not a small issue—that she was not "pleasingly plump," as she had been telling herself. This single event served as a turning point for her.

For others, getting out of the denial stage may involve more gradual realizations. They may

BOX 1: HOW BEING FAT CAN HURT YOU: POSSIBLE HAZARDS ASSOCIATED WITH OBESITY

- Coronary artery disease
- Strokes
- Diabetes mellitus
- High blood pressure
- Osteoarthritis
- Lung and breathing problems
- Complications during surgery
- Complications during childbirth
- Bone and joint pain
- Fatigue
- Low self-esteem
- Social stigmatization
- Accidents
- Physical inability to take part in some activities

ence some satisfaction, they will have to make some important decisions involving some significant changes.

Why We Stay Fat

Obesity causes many health problems (see Box 1) and can be physically and emotionally painful. However, there are (believe it or not) advantages to being overweight. The following are some of the hidden advantages of obesity—actual benefits cited by actual clients:

- "I don't have to deal with men making passes at me."
- "I can eat whatever I want to and don't have to worry."
- "If I get rejected, I can blame it on my weight and don't feel as threatened."
- "I can maintain the belief that all I have to do to improve my life is to lose weight, and I know that if I *really* wanted to, I could lose weight."
- "I get out of doing things. For instance, I can't fit behind the wheel of the car, so I don't have to drive my kids all over."

begin to realize that they are unhappy about the fact that they have to shop at special stores for their clothes, or they may begin to realize that the "postbaby" fat they are carrying around is from a baby that is now 5 years old. They may become acutely aware that the fat won't magically come off in the summer, when cantaloupe and peaches are in season. After all, they've weighed this weight for how many summers now? These realizations may culminate in the greater realization that they are unhappy with their weight and that if they wish to change the situation and experi-

Can you think of any advantages to you of being overweight? Think hard, and then list them here.

_____

_____

_____

_____

Once you become aware of some of the advantages to you of being overweight, you can begin to find effective solutions. Try to think of a way to cope with each "advantage" you listed (for example, "I can learn to be more assertive and then can deal effectively with men's passes").

_____

_____

_____

_____

_____

Where Are You in Your Stage of Weight Loss?

Many times when people decide to make life changes, they try quick fixes. An example might be an alcoholic who tries vitamin B-12 to cure alcoholism rather than trying to quit drinking. In weight loss, people use crash diets or weight-loss pills (or any number of other phony weight-loss gimmicks). They usually fail to lose weight and, in the process, lose self-confidence. Occasionally, people will lose weight with these methods. Unfortunately, long-term follow-up studies have shown that almost all people who lose weight by following anything other than a sound diet and physical activity program with behavior modification eventually regain all of their weight—and then some. When this pattern occurs repeatedly, it is called *yo-yo dieting*, and it can be very harmful.

Yo-yo dieting can be dangerous in several ways. For one thing, repeated attempts and failures at weight loss can destroy your self-confidence in your ability to successfully lose weight and keep it off. Given the fact that confidence in your ability to change seems to be very important in weight-loss success, you can see how repeated failures set you up for future failures. Also, studies have found that yo-yo dieting

can reduce your metabolic rate and, ultimately, the number of calories you spend, thus making it harder to lose weight with each new trial. Therefore, it is better never to have lost than to have lost and regained. Furthermore, when you lose weight, you generally lose fat and muscle. But when you regain weight, you regain mostly fat. Because fat burns fewer calories than muscle, this situation contributes to a reduction in metabolic rate. It also may make you appear fatter than you looked before, even at the same weight. Finally, some research suggests that yo-yo dieting increases the likelihood that you will develop heart disease. So, you can see that when you decide to lose weight, it is important to be sure that you are committed to lifelong lifestyle changes.

Further, writing down specific reasons why you want to lose weight can be a powerful motivator. Some examples of reasons people state include "I want to lose weight because my blood sugar was high at my last doctor visit, and I don't want to develop diabetes"; "I want to lose weight because many of my clothes don't fit, and I don't want to have to buy a new wardrobe"; and "I want to lose weight because I was so humiliated when I couldn't fit into that chair that I never want to feel that way again."

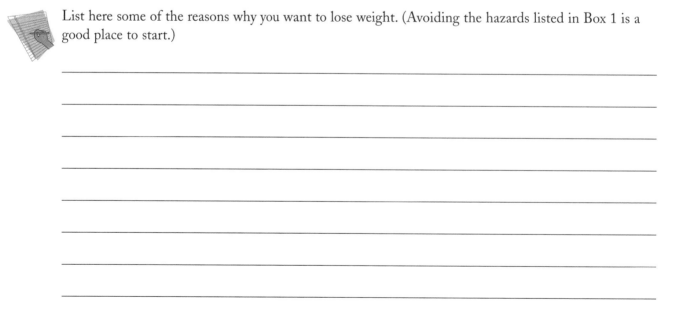

List here some of the reasons why you want to lose weight. (Avoiding the hazards listed in Box 1 is a good place to start.)

_____

_____

_____

_____

_____

_____

_____

Some people find it useful to keep this list in a visible place and to refer to it often, especially when their spirits are sagging.

Of course, wanting to lose weight is not enough. A lot of changes will be required of you. List some of the behaviors in your current lifestyle that you will need to change if you are to lose weight (for example, "I will not be able to eat butter pecan ice cream while I watch my favorite shows at night" or "I will have to set aside some time for physical activity"):

_____

_____

_____

_____

_____

_____

The Battle of the Bulge
—Are Your Weapons Drawn?

Readiness Quiz: Questions to Ask Yourself Before You Start Your Diet

Answer the following questions to assess whether or not you are ready to take the plunge:

		YES	NO
1.	Do you have a source of support for your diet and physical activity plan?	☐	☐
2.	Do you have time scheduled for physical activity?	☐	☐
3.	Have you thought about your weight history (for example, what your lowest adult weight was) and set your weight-loss goal accordingly?	☐	☐
4.	Do you believe that losing weight will improve all other areas of your life?	☐	☐
5.	Do you think that when you go off your program from time to time, you will have failed?	☐	☐
6.	Are you willing to do some self-exploration?	☐	☐
7.	If it will help you, are you willing to seek outside aid?	☐	☐
8.	Have you visualized what your life will be like when you are at your goal weight (for example, what you will have for lunch and how you will fit physical activity into your daily routine)?	☐	☐
9.	Are you willing to invest the mental energy required in learning about calories and in making daily decisions regarding your weight?	☐	☐
10.	Are you willing to keep records of your eating and physical activity until you have achieved and learned the skills of weight management?	☐	☐
11.	Do you accept the fact that weight management is a lifelong behavior and that it affects your entire life?	☐	☐
12.	Are you prepared to make weight loss one of your top priorities and to deal with adverse reactions from family members and friends at times?	☐	☐

Interpretation

Use this quiz as a guide consisting of questions to ask yourself before deciding whether you really are ready for this battle. Here are some ways to interpret your answers:

1. Do you have a source of support for your diet and physical activity plan? Research has shown that people who have a good source of support do better with both long-term and short-term weight-loss programs. Although it is best if this source of support comes, at least in part, from those you live with and are closest to, you can find support in other places. This step is an important one to take before starting a weight-loss program.

2. Do you have time scheduled for physical activity? Your answer to this question serves a couple of purposes. First, it tells you whether you have thought about the practical considerations involved in weight loss, such as when you will fit in your physical activity. Second, it tells you whether or not you recognize the critical role physical activity plays in long-term weight management and are willing to act accordingly.

3. Have you thought about your weight history and set your weight-loss goal accordingly? Many people with weight problems have a long history of failure when it comes to weight loss. One contributing factor is setting unrealistic goals. For instance, if your lowest adult weight was 150 pounds when you were 20 years old and you have weighed 200 pounds for 25 years, a goal weight of 120 pounds is probably not realistic. Could you be happy at a higher goal weight under these circumstances? Considering past successes and what was helpful in achieving them is also important. If you found that you were better able to follow a diet when you didn't travel to work, you may need to focus extra effort on a "commuting strategy." Likewise, if you know that you will not give up sweets, find a way to fit them into a nutritious, low-calorie plan.

4. Do you believe that losing weight will improve all other areas of your life? Feeling better about yourself will improve your health, can improve your self-image, and may improve your marriage or relationships with others. However, there is no guarantee that losing weight will drastically improve your life much at all. You may find that your spouse finds other ways to criticize you or that you are as shy as you always have been. Recognize that weight loss will probably improve your quality of life, but it will not fix everything.

5. Do you think that when you go off your program from time to time, you will have failed? Weight management is a lifelong process and must be viewed as such. No one can be perfect for a whole lifetime. If you expect to be perfect, you are setting yourself up for a failure down the road. A more realistic and helpful approach is to set realistic goals each day, and to allow breathing room for days when you will not be perfect.

6. Are you willing to do some self-exploration? A well-respected psychologist conducted a nationwide survey to find out if there were any advantages to being overweight. What he learned was surprising. Many of the people he surveyed identified advantages to being overweight. For example, some women were afraid that if they were at a desirable weight, they would cheat on their husbands.* Other advantages of being overweight include feeling protected, having an excuse not to perform certain activities, and not having to talk to people. Without recognizing such issues, you cannot begin to solve your weight problem.

7. If it will help you, are you willing to seek outside aid? Sometimes, it is necessary to resolve other problems before you can be ready to lose weight. One woman went through counseling while undergoing a weight-loss program. She said that as a result of counseling, she learned to be more assertive and to place her needs first. She has been able to maintain her weight for several years now, in part because she was better prepared to deal with the emotional issues that can interfere with weight management.

*R. Stuart and B. Jacobson. *Weight, Sex and Marriage: A Delicate Balance.* New York, NY: Norton; 1991.

8. *Have you visualized what your life will be like when you are at your goal weight?* Maintaining a lower body weight involves some sacrifices. It may require you to drastically reduce your intake of favorite foods. It may well mean spending less time at home doing what you want and more time at the gym exercising. It means making decisions on a regular basis regarding your calorie intake. It may mean doing away with the traditional Friday night banana splits and going for a small fat-free frozen yogurt instead. Have you thought about these things? Are you ready for them?

9. *Are you willing to invest the mental energy required in learning about calories and in making daily decisions regarding your weight?* You would not fantasize that you could stay within your financial budget without looking at prices. Why would you think you could stay within your calorie budget without looking at calories? To learn about calories requires time and effort. You will have to become aware of portion sizes and read up on calories. This method is the best way to know the wisest choices regarding your diet. By learning which foods are high in calories and which are low, you increase your options and likelihood of success. This process is time-consuming at first, but as you learn calorie counts, you can gradually reduce the time required and gain more independence.

10. *Are you willing to keep records of your eating and physical activity until you have achieved and learned the skills of weight management?* Most people don't write checks without recording the amount in a check register. The only way to be sure that you have a balanced budget is to write down your deposits and withdrawals. Research has shown that the best way to ensure a calorie deficit (weight loss) is to do the same thing with what you eat (deposits) and what you spend in physical activity (withdrawals). This activity is time-consuming and requires a lot of commitment. However, it has been found to be one of the most effective techniques for ensuring weight loss.

11. *Do you accept that fact that weight management is a lifelong behavior and that it affects your entire life?* Successful weight managers recognize that weight loss and weight management are lifelong processes. They have no beginning or end. The dietary choices necessary to lose weight are the same as the choices required to maintain that loss. Although the process does get easier, it does not end.

12. *Are you prepared to make weight loss one of your top priorities and to deal at times with adverse reactions from family members and friends?* One of the hardest parts of weight loss is that it often competes with other demands. Women are especially vulnerable to this problem, because they tend to place the needs of others above their own. Sometimes, close friends or family members will sabotage your efforts. They may take it personally when you no longer wish to partake in the Friday night banana split. They may not understand why you don't want to bake chocolate chip cookies anymore. Making weight loss a priority also means that when you are tired, you still will have to go exercise even though you would rather sleep. These issues can make weight loss extra difficult. Are you ready to tackle these challenges?

Principles of Weight Loss

Obesity has existed for a very long time. Cave drawings of obese human figures have been reported. Millennia-old fertility figurines depict obese versions of females (known as Venus figures), made during a time when obesity had survival value. But never in human history (to our knowledge) has the incidence of obesity been as great as it is today. Experts in recent years have accumulated strong evidence supporting the role of genetics in human obesity. Vigorous efforts are under way to develop "anti-obesity" drugs. In years to come, books such as this one may be obsolete. In the meantime, however, you still need to know some facts.

Reasons for Obesity

First of all, even if you do have "fat genes," your obesity is probably caused by a combination of genetics, environment, and psychosocial issues. These factors explain why so much obesity exists in the United States today, when high-fat diets and sedentary lifestyles are the norm.

Fast food is a multimillion-dollar industry, and there is fierce competition among the chains for your dollar. This fact translates into a constant bombardment of food advertisements and bigger meal deals (meaning more fat and calories for your money). And it isn't just the fast-food industry that is working against you and trying to steal your skinny dreams away. Many food companies are trying to entice you. The advertisements are on billboards, in magazines, on television, and on the radio. Every time your eyes come across a food ad, you are reminded that there are all kinds of different, delicious flavors waiting for you. You may not even be thinking about a char-grilled hamburger with sharp cheddar cheese; rich, creamy mayonnaise; and fresh lettuce and tomatoes all on a lightly toasted sesame seed bun.

However, after you hear a commercial that vividly describes the tasty food, you find that you can't get it off your mind. That's when you cave in and drive through Burger Breakthrough. This sort of advertising, which serves as a daily threat to weight loss, is difficult to avoid. Further, because fat tastes good, manufacturers create high-fat (and thus high-calorie) foods—fat sells. This fact also contributes to the obesity epidemic.

Besides genes and environmental factors, psychosocial factors also influence weight. For example, a problem frequently encountered in this country is loneliness. Many people say that food is their best friend. How can you just let go of your best friend?

Also, people today live in a high-stress world. Again, you can always count on food to be there. (The food industry will see to that!) When you have a deadline, you may not feel you have time to go for a walk or take a hot bath. But you can eat cookies while you work. Another example of how psychosocial issues affect weight is that being overweight is actually advantageous in some situations, as already discussed. Many more examples of how people use food to cope will be supplied throughout the text.

Basics of Weight Loss

Regardless of the fact that environmental and psychosocial factors may keep people fat, you still need to know the basics about weight loss. Think of it this way: Can you balance your checkbook if you don't know what your deposits, withdrawals, and checking account charges are? Can you find the best deals on purchases if you never look at prices? In the same fashion, it is necessary to learn basic information about the factors that influence your weight. Here are the facts:

- It takes 3,500 calories to gain or lose 1 pound of body fat.
- To gain 1 pound of fat, you must take in (deposit) 3,500 calories more than you burn (withdraw).
- To lose 1 pound of fat, you must burn (withdraw) 3,500 calories more than you take in (deposit).
- You take in calories by eating and drinking.
- You burn calories in your everyday life by the work of living (breathing, digesting food, pumping blood, and so on), through activities of daily living (walking from the car to a building, making the bed, getting up to answer the phone, and so forth), and through physical activity.

You cannot influence the number of calories your body burns through the work of living, but you can influence the calories your body burns in your activities of daily living and in physical activity. Of course, you also can influence the calories you take in by selecting lower-calorie foods and by eating less. To give you an idea of what is involved, Table 1 lists sample calorie contents. Table 2 lists calorie expenditures on various physical activities.

Muscle burns more calories than fat. This fact means that pound for pound, a lean, muscular person will burn more calories than a fat person. However, fat people may require more total calories, because they have more pounds to burn calories. As you lose weight, your total calorie requirement may drop, because your total weight will be less. Therefore, physical activity is very important in weight loss, because it burns calories and helps you lose weight. Physical activity also

TABLE 1: CALORIES IN SELECTED FOODS

Food	Calories
1 Hershey's Kiss	25
1 chili dog	320
1 Big Mac	570
3-piece fried fish dinner	1,180
1 medium apple	100
1 fig bar	45
1 tablespoon butter	100
1 tablespoon sugar	50
6-ounce steak	600
6 ounces of broiled shrimp	150

burns calories when you are maintaining weight, and it may make the difference between your having to follow a 1,500-calorie diet or an 1,800-calorie diet. Which would you rather live on?

Obtaining Initial Weights and Measurements

When beginning a weight-loss program, first determine your starting point. The most basic way is to learn your weight. Some basic guidelines to follow:

1. Always weigh yourself first thing in the morning, before you eat or drink anything. At this time of day you will obtain the most accurate weight. If you drink a 16-ounce soda and then weigh yourself a half hour later, you will weigh 1 pound more, because you will have that extra pound of fluid in your body. It's that straightforward.

TABLE 2: CALORIES BURNED PER MINUTE, BY INDIVIDUAL'S WEIGHT

ACTIVITY	120 POUNDS	140 POUNDS	160 POUNDS	180 POUNDS	200 POUNDS	220 POUNDS
Aerobic dance	5.7	6.6	7.5	8.5	9.4	10.3
Walking (4 miles per hour)	4.7	5.5	6.3	7.1	7.8	8.6
Jogging (11-minute mile)	8.4	9.8	11.2	12.6	14.0	15.4
Bicycling (13 miles per hour)	9.1	10.5	11.9	13.3	14.7	16.0

2. Always weigh yourself on the same scale. Some scales weigh lighter or heavier than others, so it's best to use the same scale for consistency.

3. Measurements are very useful. As you start exercising, you may add muscle while you lose fat. As a result, your actual weight loss will be less than you might expect, though your fat loss may be good. Measurements will reflect these changes.

4. Your body mass index (BMI) is a calculation of your weight relative to your height. Calculate your BMI as follows:

   Multiply your weight (in pounds) by 703.

   Divide that number by your height (in inches).

   Divide that new number by your height (in inches) again.

   In other words, weight × 703 ÷ height ÷ height = BMI.

Say you weigh 210 pounds and are 62 inches tall. 210 × 703 ÷ 62 ÷ 62 = BMI of 38. A BMI of 25 to 29.9 means you are overweight, and a BMI of 30 or more means you are obese (see Box 2). When determining a goal weight, consider your BMI, but also consider your weight history.

BOX 2: EVALUATING YOUR BODY MASS INDEX (BMI)

Weight Classification	BMI
Underweight	Below 18.5
Normal	18.5–24.9
Overweight	25.0–29.9
Obese	30.0 and above

Source: National Heart, Lung, and Blood Institute. Aim for a healthy weight.
Available at: http://www.nhlbi.nih.gov/health/public/heart/obesity/lose_wt/risk.htm. Accessed April 26, 2003.

What is the lowest weight you have been in adulthood? How much physical activity are you willing to do? How hard are you willing to work? Losing small amounts of weight can result in big improvements in health. BMI does not measure body fat, however, and results can be misleading for people with unusually muscular or lean builds. It is possible to have a high BMI without having excess fat. Skin-fold calipers measure fat under the skin and can be an accurate way to measure body fat if used by a trained professional.

Nutrition and Weight Loss

The goal of weight loss is to look and feel better. Have you ever tried the diet-soda-and-sugarless-gum diet? You can always spot people on that diet—they are the ones who are obsessing about food, have big bags under their eyes, and don't have the energy to tear open a packet of artificial sweetener. They neither look nor feel better, even if their clothes are looser.

The only way to lose weight and keep it off while maintaining your health is to eat a balanced diet with at least three meals a day. Believe it or not, studies on weight-loss maintainers found that one of the things they had in common was that they ate breakfast! Eating a variety of foods from all food groups can help you lose weight without weakening your bones, causing kidney disease, or doing any other damage to your body. The Food Guide Pyramid (Figure 1) shows how many servings from each food group you should try to eat each day. Skimping can actually slow down weight loss and increase muscle loss, making it harder to maintain your new weight.

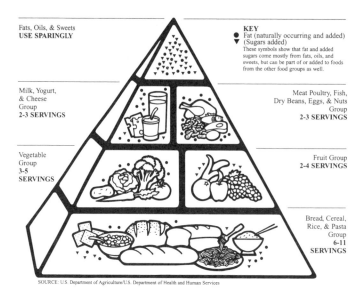

Figure 1: The Food Guide Pyramid

How Many Calories Can You Eat and Still Lose Weight?

Calorie needs vary and will be affected by your weight, height, age, activity level, gender, and musculature; certain medications; and other factors. The best way to determine your actual calorie needs is with a calorimeter—a large, technically sophisticated piece of equipment that measures calorie expenditure. Most people don't have access to such equipment and generally don't need to use one. They can find a calorie level that will be appropriate for weight loss by multiplying their weight (in pounds) by 10 to 12. The resulting total generally ranges between 1,200 calories (for small, older, and moderately overweight women) and 2,000 calories (for larger, younger males). This calculation can give you a starting place for your weight-loss program without reducing your calorie intake to ineffectively low levels.

Meal Patterns for Healthy Weight Loss

Table 3 lists meal patterns for calorie levels ranging from 1,200 calories to 2,000 calories.

FRUIT SERVINGS

One serving of fruit equals the following:

- 1 small banana, apple, mango, or orange
- 17 grapes
- 1 medium peach
- 2 small plums
- 1 cup raspberries
- 1 cup honeydew melon cubes
- ½ cup juice
- ½ cup unsweetened canned fruit
- ¼ cup dried fruit

NONSTARCHY VEGETABLE SERVINGS

One serving of nonstarchy vegetables equals the following:

- ½ cup cooked vegetables
- ½ cup vegetable juice
- 1 cup raw vegetables

LEAN MEAT AND MEAT SUBSTITUTE SERVINGS

One serving of lean meat or meat substitute equals the following:

- 1 ounce water-packed tuna
- 1 ounce white-meat chicken
- 1 ounce lean luncheon meat
- ½ cup cooked beans, peas, or lentils
- 1 ounce lean round steak or sirloin
- 1 ounce pork tenderloin
- 1 ounce low-fat cheese

TABLE 3: MEAL PATTERNS FOR HEALTHY WEIGHT LOSS					
	1,200 Calories	1,400 Calories	1,600 Calories	1,800 Calories	2,000 Calories
Fruit servings	2	2	3	3	3
Nonstarchy vegetable servings	3	3	3–4	4	4
Lean meat or meat substitute servings	6	6	6	6	6
Bread/starch servings	6	6	7	9	10
Fat-free dairy servings	2	2	2	2	2
Fat servings	2	2	3	3	4
Free-food calories	—	150	200	200–250	250

Source: Adapted with permission from American Dietetic Association/American Diabetes Association, *Exchange Lists for Weight Management,* 2003.

BREAD/STARCH SERVINGS

One serving of bread/starch equals the following:

- ⅓ cup cooked pasta
- ½ cup potatoes
- ⅓ cup cooked rice
- ½ cup cooked beans, peas, and lentils
- 1 medium slice bread (1 ounce)
- ½ (1-ounce) hot dog or hamburger bun
- 3 cups popped low-fat or no-fat-added popcorn
- ½ cup cooked cereal
- ¾ cup unsweetened ready-to-eat cereal

FAT-FREE DAIRY SERVINGS

One serving of fat-free dairy equals the following:

- 1 cup fat-free milk
- 6 ounces artificially sweetened, fat-free yogurt

FAT SERVINGS

One serving of fat equals the following:

- 1 teaspoon margarine, butter, or oil
- 1 slice bacon

FREE FOOD

Calories for free food can be spent on any food at all. Just limit the calories from these foods to the number of calories allowed. Foods such as lettuce, green pepper, bean sprouts, onion, and cucumber can be eaten without restriction. Diet soda, diet lemonade, artificial sweeteners, and sugar-free gelatin desserts also can be consumed in unrestricted amounts, though moderate intake is recommended. Mustard, vinegar, hot sauce, and lemon juice can be used in unlimited amounts.

FAST FOODS

Dining out has become an integral part of the American way of life. Although it is easy to overdose on calories when eating out, it is not inevitable. Knowing how to order will allow you to eat out, even at fast-food restaurants, while sticking with your weight-loss or weight-maintenance plan. Table 4 (page 14) lists many fast-food options and their calorie counts.

TABLE 4: **FAST-FOOD RESTAURANT GUIDE**

Food	Calories
Burger King	
Hamburger	310
Original Whopper Sandwich	710
Chicken Tenders, 5 pieces	210
Onion rings, medium order	320
Shake, vanilla, small	560
McDonald's	
Big Mac	590
Filet-O-Fish	470
French fries, small	210
French fries, super size	610
Egg McMuffin	300
Subway	
Club, 6 inch	320
Roast beef, 6 inch	290
Turkey breast, 6 inch	280
Meatball, 6 inch	530
Taco Bell	
7-Layer Burrito	530
Grilled Stuft Burrito, chicken	680
Nachos	320
Cheese quesadilla	490
Soft taco, beef	210
KFC	
Breast, no skin or breading	140
Breast, Original Recipe	380
Breast, Extra Crispy	460
Breast, Hot & Spicy	460
Biscuit	180
Mashed potatoes and gravy	120
Pizza Hut	
Veggie Lover's, Thin 'N Crispy, 1 small slice	190
Italian Sausage, Thin 'N Crispy, 1 small slice	290
Meat Lover's, Pan, 1 small slice	340
Cheese, Stuffed Crust, 1 small slice	360

Source: Companies' Web sites, accessed April 18, 2003.

Common Weight-Loss Myths to Keep You Fat

The following list of weight-loss myths includes actual (but unverified) claims made in the past in popular dieting books, as well as "unofficial" beliefs that people may harbor, even if they are not aware of them:

Myth

Myth: Grapefruit, celery, and _____ (fill in the blank) actually burn more calories than they contain.

Myth: You should eat foods from only one food group at any meal, because your body can't handle digesting all the different food types at once.

Myth: Broken cookies don't have calories, because they have all leaked out.

Myth: If you want to lose weight in your stomach, do sit-ups; if you want to lose weight in your thighs, do leg-lifts; and so on.

Myth: If I just watch my fat intake, I can lose weight.

Myth: Cleaning your plate is a social responsibility (children are starving in Africa).

Fact

Fact: There are no negative-calorie foods. If you eat enough grapefruit, you will gain weight.

Fact: When you eat, a few body organs are involved in digestion and automatically secrete enzymes for this job. The digestive tract is perfectly capable of digesting a variety of foods at any given time, and the body is capable of handling and storing the end products of digestion as well.

Fact: Even small bites of foods have calories.

Fact: You cannot determine from which part of your body you will lose weight. When you lose weight, you usually lose it all over. Doing sit-ups can help to tone your stomach muscles, but if there is too much fat on your stomach, you won't be able to see your muscles anyhow.

Fact: This statement may be true if following a low-fat diet reduces your calorie intake enough. However, calories are still the bottom line for weight loss (and reducing fat intake is the first step in reducing calorie intake).

Fact: Cleaning your plate doesn't do starving people any good (and meanwhile, people are getting fat in the United States). If you want to help, prepare less food and send the money you save to charity.

"How Much Does It Cost?"
—*Determining Calories in Foods*

Everyone knows that a necessary part of weight loss is calorie reduction. One way to reduce calorie intake is to eat less food. Another important approach is to learn which foods are lowest in calories in the first place. If you pick low-calorie foods, you will find you can have more food by volume.

For example, say that you are trying to eat your protein, so you eat a piece of prime rib. If this prime rib is 12 ounces, you will have eaten 1,200 calories. In contrast, if you were aware of calories, you would realize that you could have met your protein requirements by eating 6 ounces of broiled snapper for 150 calories, leaving enough room for a tossed salad, 1 cup of green vegetables, a 6-ounce baked potato, 2 tablespoons of fat-free dressing, a 1-ounce dinner roll, ½ cup fat-free frozen yogurt, and a diet soda. After all is said and done, you would have eaten less than 500 calories (versus 1,200), while eating more food, and you probably would feel more satisfied. This example shows why it is helpful to know where the calories are in foods: if you know, you can make the best choices.

Where Do Calories Come From?

Why does prime rib have so many more calories than broiled flounder? Before you can begin to understand the answer, you must learn a little bit about where the calories in foods come from. Basically, calories in the diet come from four different places: *carbohydrates, proteins, alcohol,* and *fat*. Carbohydrates, proteins, and fats are called *macronutrients*, because they are eaten in large amounts compared with vitamins and minerals (which are called *micronutrients*). Each of these energy-providing macronutrients makes a different calorie contribution to your diet:

- Carbohydrates provide 4 calories per gram.
- Proteins provide 4 calories per gram.
- Alcohol provides 7 calories per gram.
- Fats provide 9 calories per gram.

Repeat: fats provide 9 calories! Per gram! That means that fats provide more than twice as many calories per gram as either carbohydrates or proteins. This fact explains why prime rib and other fatty foods pack in the calories. Another way to look at this comparison is that 1 tablespoon of a pure carbohydrate (say, sugar) has 50 calories, whereas 1 tablespoon of a pure fat (say, oil) has 120 calories. You could have more than 2 tablespoons of carbohydrate for every tablespoon of fat. Once again, when you cut back on your fat calories, you can eat more total food volume. For example, you can have 4 ounces of baked flounder for the same number of calories as 1 ounce of prime rib. You can have 2 slices of bread versus half of a biscuit. You can have 1 cup of fat-free, sugar-free frozen yogurt versus ⅙ cup of gelato. Do you get the idea?

In addition to the fact that excess dietary fat adds excess calories, diets high in fat have been linked with heart disease and cancer, and possibly other diseases as well.

Water Wonders

The discussion of calories does not end here with carbohydrates, proteins, alcohol, and fat. Another dietary factor influences calorie levels in foods. This factor is *water*. Water does not provide calories, but it does add *volume*. Take, for instance, 15 grapes versus 15 raisins. What's the crucial difference between them? The grapes have water, but the raisins (dehydrated grapes) do not. Therefore, you can place the relatively large grapes in a bowl and eat them one at a time, in 15 bites. The raisins, in contrast, can be eaten in one fell swoop. If you are having a snack, which would be more satisfying: 1 bite or 15 bites? Here is another example: Many people are surprised to learn that one 3-ounce fat-free bagel has 240 calories. They wonder why, if the bagel doesn't have any fat or sugar, does it have so many calories? The answer is that it doesn't have any moisture to dilute the calories. Think about dry rice versus cooked rice: ¼ cup of dry rice contains 200 calories, and 1 cup of cooked rice also contains 200 calories. Why the difference? You got it: water!

Examining Food Labels

When buying prepackaged foods, you have probably noticed the food labels. Manufacturers are required by law to give a nutritional breakdown of all foods, with a few exceptions, on the package (see Figure 2).

Nutrition Facts

Serving Size: 1/2 muffin
Servings Per Container: 2

Amount Per Serving

Calories 220	Calories from Fat 110

	%Daily Value*
Total Fat 12g	**18%**
Saturated Fat 6g	**30%**
Cholesterol 0mg	**0%**
Sodium 330mg	**14%**
Total Carbohydrate 25g	**8%**
Dietary Fiber Less Than 1g	**4%**
Sugars 12g	
Protein 2g	

Vitamin A 2%	●	Vitamin C 0%
Calcium 4%	●	Iron 6%

*Percent daily values are based on a 2,000-calorie diet. Your daily values may be higher or lower, depending on your calorie needs:

	Calories:	2,000	2,500
Total Fat	Less than	65g	80g
Saturated Fat	Less than	20g	25g
Cholesterol	Less than	300mg	300mg
Sodium	Less than	2,400mg	2,400mg
Total Carbohydrate		300g	375g
Dietary Fiber		25g	30g

Calories per Gram:

Fat 9	●	Carbohydrate 4	●	Protein 4

Figure 2: Food Label

Here is the information you need to keep in mind as you study a food label:

■ Look for serving size. Information is listed *per serving, not per container.* So if you eat more than one serving, you need to do the math to know how many calories, how many fat grams, and how much sodium you will be eating. It is a good idea to think about these things before you buy a food. For example, if the label on a muffin package says that it has 220 calories per serving and that there are two servings per container (even though it's only one muffin), that means the whole muffin will have 440 calories. If you know you always eat the whole container when you buy one, think about how many calories you will be taking in before you buy it. A smaller container may be better, even if it costs more.

■ Read the labels of different foods to determine the best buy in terms of calorie cost. And just because a food is labeled "low fat," "low sugar," or whatever doesn't mean it will work on your weight-loss plan. Look at the calories per serving.

■ The information listed in the "% Daily Value" column is based on a 2,000-calorie diet. If your meal plan contains fewer or more calories, these percentages will not apply to you as they are stated.

■ For the sake of health, try to keep your total fat intake to less than 30 percent of your calories. For most people on a calorie-restricted diet, that total is about 45 grams to 50 grams of fat per day. You can see from the sample label in Figure 2 that one food item can easily meet a substantial portion of your daily fat allowance, and in some cases all of it. This whole muffin provides 24 grams of fat (about 50 percent of the daily recommendation). Most of the fat you consume should be from monounsaturated sources. Limit saturated fats (mostly found in fatty meats, whole milk, and whole-milk dairy products) and *trans* fatty acids (found in hydrogenated oils, such as the fat in commercially baked products, margarines, and shortening).

This discussion of calories should help you to understand and make better food choices, even when you don't know the exact calorie contents of foods. But if you are serious about losing weight, a calorie book is crucial. Dieting without a calorie book is like shopping on a budget without knowing prices. Several calorie books are available in bookstores. One pocket-sized version is *The T-Factor Fat Gram Counter*, by Jamie Pope and Martin Katahn (New York: Norton, 1999). Another book is *Bowes and Church's Food Values of Portions Commonly Used*, by Jean Pennington (Philadelphia, Pa: Lippincott, 1998). This book is too big to carry around, but it is more comprehensive. Labels are also an excellent source of calorie information, and many chain restaurants now offer nutrition information upon request. However, when using these sources for information, it is always important to look at the serving sizes. Many calorie books do not provide specific serving sizes, and the calorie counts they list can deviate significantly from actual calorie values of portions you eat.

Mapping Out Your Course

It is difficult to find directions if you don't have a specific destination in mind. Just as you must know where you want to go before you turn on the engine of your car and start to drive, so you must know what you want to achieve before you embark upon life-changing programs. Goals serve the purpose of letting you know what your destination is. When you have a goal in mind, you can develop a plan for reaching it. Goals serve other functions, too. They help you make a commitment to a behavior change. They also help you stay focused on the direction you want to head. Goals are especially helpful if you write them down and post them in a few visible places where you will see them several times a day (for example, on your bathroom mirror, in your car, on the refrigerator, and at your desk at work).

Goal Setting

Although goal setting sounds easy enough, inappropriate goals can set you up for failure. If you want to set goals that will help you succeed, here are some guidelines:

1. Goals should be realistic. If your ultimate goal is to lose 50 pounds, you should not aim to lose it in, say, 2 months. That time frame is unrealistic and is a setup for failure. Many dieters do this to themselves. They set goals that are difficult or impossible to achieve. Then, when they fail, they reinforce the belief that there is something wrong with themselves, that they are inherently incapable of losing weight, that they have no willpower, and so on. This belief only makes it harder to adhere to a weight-loss plan, and it is not constructive. When you set goals, they should be both challenging and realistic at the same time.

2. Goals should be progressive. This rule is in keeping with the first rule—that goals should be realistic. It is sometimes helpful to break down your ultimate goal into several small goals. For instance, if your ultimate goal is to walk for 30 minutes five times a week, you may break it down and start with 5 minutes two times a week. This provides you with a more manageable goal and is not as overwhelming. It also allows you to experience mini-successes and reinforces the fact that you can indeed stick to an exercise plan and change your behaviors in a healthy way. As long as you continue to set more goals based on your most recent successes, you will get to your ultimate goal step by step, one step at a time.

3. **Goals should be specific.** When setting goals, always know very clearly what you want. If your goal is to lose weight, state exactly how many pounds you want to lose; if your goal is to improve your eating habits, state specifically how you want to improve your eating habits. For example, a specific goal of how you would like to improve your eating habits might be as follows: "I will improve my eating habits by eating five fruits and vegetables each day, including one high in vitamin A and one high in vitamin C."

4. **Goals should have specific start dates and accomplish dates.** Determining these dates will help you commit yourself to a time frame and get off the "I'll start on Monday" track. For example, you might write your goal as follows: "For the first week of June, I will eat salad before I eat a high-calorie snack."

5. **Goals should be in writing.** Studies show that successful people often have written goals. Writing it down makes a goal more visible and tangible. It also helps you make a commitment to the goal. When goals are in writing, you can post them in places to serve as reminders. See page 21 for an example of how a sample contract can be completed (Box 3) and a form that you can complete (Box 4).

6. **Goals should be flexible.** Having flexible goals does not mean that you should change a goal every time it gets challenging or difficult. What it means is that you can decide that your goal is a bad goal or that it is not really a goal at all, and you then can change it. For example, say your goal is to exercise three mornings a week before you go to work. If, at the end of the week, you realize that you did not reach your goal because you kept hitting the snooze button and going back to sleep, you need to reassess your goal. Decide if it is a goal you really want to accomplish, or if you can reach the same end point in a different way. If you still want to try to achieve your initial goal of exercising in the morning, you may need to step back and decide on a strategy to help you get out of bed in the morning. You could move the alarm clock to the other side of the room, go to bed earlier, or use other creative strategies. Whatever you do, do not assume that you are at fault. If you are having trouble reaching a particular goal, the goal may be faulty and may need to be revised.

7. **Weekly goals should be behavioral.** Once you have decided on a goal weight and on a reasonable amount of time in which you want to lose the weight, any other goals you set should be goals over which you have direct control. You can't directly influence how much weight you will lose this week, because you may retain fluid one day or hit a plateau. So you should not word your goal as "Lose 2 pounds this week." This can set you up to fail. You can control the behaviors that lead to weight loss, however (for example, how many calories you eat, drink, and spend with physical activities). Therefore, your goals should be based on *behaviors*—things you can directly control.

Goal-Setting Exercise

Bear in mind the golden rules of goal setting you just learned as you go through the following exercise.

First, think about what your ultimate weight goal is. List it here: _____

Next, think about the kind of lifestyle you will be required to lead to get to and maintain this weight. For instance, if your ultimate weight goal is 130 pounds, are you willing to exercise aerobically five times per week and eat 1,800 calories per day for the rest of your life to maintain that weight, or would the lifestyle associated with a weight of 160 pounds be more acceptable to you?

Next, decide on a realistic time frame for reaching this goal. (Remember that it takes a deficit of 3,500 calories to lose 1 pound.)

Fill in the following: I would like to reach my ultimate weight goal of _____ pounds by _____. (This is a general time frame, because you do not have direct control over the pounds you lose—only the behaviors that lead to weight loss.)

Have you thought about what will be required of you to accomplish this goal? How

many calories a day will you be allowed? What will this number translate into in terms of meals? Are there any holidays or celebrations coming up that might interrupt your plans or for which you might want to allow some extra calories? Think about these things when you establish your goal. This planning is part of setting yourself up for success.

Once you have a solid goal in mind and a realistic time frame, put this goal in writing, and sign your name to it. It may even be helpful to have someone else cosign it.

Finally, decide on a plan of action, and establish some behavioral goals. For example, if you realize that you want to lose 1 pound per week, you know you will have to remove 500 calories per day from your life to accomplish this. This will allow you to establish an approximate daily calorie level. Some examples of behavioral goals that might help you stay within your desired calorie level include keeping washed, sliced carrots and celery in the refrigerator at all times for snacks; going for a walk, either indoors or outside, before eating lunch; and developing five low-calorie lunch and dinner menus.

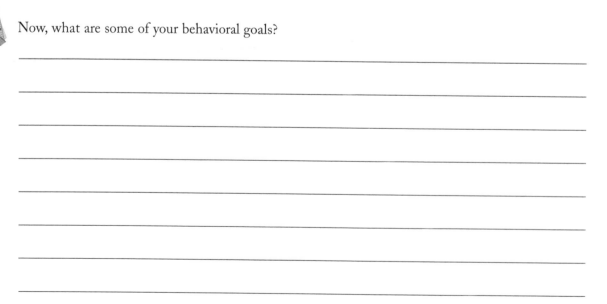

Now, what are some of your behavioral goals?

_____

_____

_____

_____

_____

_____

_____

_____

Putting these goals in writing will help you remember your game plan. Post these goals in visible places to remind you of the strategies you have developed. Appendix A and Appendix B include forms for recording and tracking your progress.

BOX 3: SAMPLE CONTRACT

I, _____John Doe_____, commit to the following goal as of _____6/6_____:

I will limit my intake of potato chips to 2 ounces per week. _____

Steps I will take to reach this goal include the following:

1. Not going to the chips section when I buy gas. _____
2. Not going to the vending machine at work. _____
3. Not keeping chips in the house. _____

_____   _____
Signature   Date

_____   _____
Witness's Signature   Date

BOX 4: CONTRACT

I, _____, commit to the following goal as of _____:

_____

_____

_____

_____

Steps I will take to reach this goal include the following:

1. _____

2. _____

3. _____

4. _____

5. _____

_____   _____
Signature   Date

_____   _____
Witness's Signature   Date

Put It in Writing!
—Self-monitoring

Many dieters have a pretty good idea of what they eat. Maybe you ate cereal and milk for breakfast; a sandwich for lunch; and fish, potatoes, and peas for dinner. Oh, and a dish of ice cream for a snack. If you add up the calories, they're 100 calories for the cereal, 100 for the milk, 150 for the bread, 200 for the lunch meat, 150 for the fish, 75 for the potatoes, 50 for the peas, and 175 for the ice cream. The total for this day is 1,000 calories (as a rough estimate). Based on this estimate, it just doesn't seem fair: Why can't you lose weight when you are eating only 1,000 calories per day? Well, if you had a fantastic memory, you might look back and realize that what you *really* had was 1½ cups of cereal at 165 calories; 1½ cups of milk at 150; milk and sugar in your coffee at 35; 1 piece of a broken cookie at 55; 1 package of peanut butter crackers at 220; a sandwich with 2 pieces of bread, lunch meat, and mayonnaise at 500 calories (versus the 350 you remembered at first); a handful of chips at 75; 2 cups of coffee with half-and-half and sugar at 100; 2 pieces of hard candy at 50; 6 ounces of baked fish with a dab of margarine (a "dab" being 1 table-spoon) at 250; 1 cup of potatoes with margarine at 250; ½ cup of peas with 1 teaspoon of margarine at 110; a Coke at 150; 4 saltines at 50; and 1 cup of reg-ular ice cream at 330 calories (or 1 cup of Haagen-Dazs at 600). The total, based on this more accurate recall, is 2,490 calories (or 2,760 if you had Haagen-Dazs). Wouldn't this tally help you understand your "plateau" a little bit better? The point is that when you write things down, you are getting an honest, realistic picture of what you are doing. This process helps you in many ways.

Why Write Down What You Eat?

Writing down what you eat has many advantages:

1. It allows you to see your eating habits. You may think that you are eating only 1,000 calories a day and really can't understand why you aren't losing weight. You might get discouraged with your failed attempts at weight loss, thinking that you have "bad genes" and will never realize your goal. Getting a picture of what you are really eating may let you know otherwise.

2. Once you have a realistic picture of what you are doing, you can identify your dietary prob-lems. For instance, in the previous example of a day's calorie intake, if you go back and review the *accurate* food records, you might realize that a lot of calories could be saved by using Molly McButter instead of margarine, using mustard instead of mayonnaise, and finding a dif-ferent evening snack. By becoming aware and making these three changes, you can save more than 600 calories—calories you did not even realize you were taking in.

3. Keeping track of what you eat, when you eat it, also increases your awareness. In the pre-vious example, if you had been keeping track of food as you ate it, you would have realized that you were eating foods that you didn't even think about. Snacks such as a piece of a cookie, hard candy at the desk, and a "little handful of chips" can really add up in a day. Yet if you don't write them down, they don't seem to count. Putting them in writing makes you see how much they really do count.

4. Writing food down as you eat it also makes you confront what you are doing and decide hon-estly whether eating it is something you really want to do after all. In the previous example, maybe if you had been forced to write down the package of peanut butter crackers along with the 220 calories it included, you

would have chosen diet soda instead. People often choose to stay in "denial" about their behaviors because they don't want to face the fact that they are betraying themselves. In the end, though, the consequences of the behavior become apparent, and they have to face them anyhow. If you simply confront your eating behaviors by writing down what you eat *when you eat it*, then at least you can make an honest decision about what you want to do.

5. Keeping track of what you eat can help you track your progress. It also can help you see in writing whether or not you are meeting your goals. It is a good idea to keep your old food records. They will help you see where you came from and thus help you during times when you get discouraged. They also can explain things, such as why you didn't gain weight last month but are gaining weight this month. You also can use successful days or weeks as a model for future behavior. For instance, if you went to a wedding in the past and practiced good dieting skills, you can review that day to recall what you did to make it successful.

6. Writing down what you eat, along with the calorie content of each food, helps you learn the calories in foods. As you learn calorie contents, you will be able to keep records in less time and will be less reliant on calorie books and scales and become more independent with your weight loss.

7. Keeping food records can help you identify your behavior patterns and give you some information for problem solving. For example, if you keep track of the mood you are in, the people you are with, and the time you eat (and any other information you think might be important), then you can identify circumstances that lead to either success or failure. You may decide that you would rather avoid a certain person while you are trying to lose weight, that you need to develop some healthy ways to cope with sadness, or that you should allow more calories for your evening snack. Information about your eating patterns can help you determine where to take action.

Feelings about Food Records

Keeping food records is strongly associated with success in weight loss, as many studies on dieting have shown. Why, then, do so many dieters choose not to keep these records? Some people don't keep food records because the activity is tedious. One way to combat this problem is to keep your records and a pen on hand at all times. Other people don't want to keep track of what they eat because they believe it takes the fun out of eating. Something happens to that devious sense of fun that goes with eating a banana split when you have to calculate and confront the fact that it has 1,500 calories. Part of the way self-monitoring works, though, is by forcing you to pay attention to your behavior today so that you won't have to avoid the scale tomorrow.

Take a few minutes to think about how you feel about food records by answering these questions:

Do you like keeping food records? _____

Why do you feel that way? _____

_____

_____

Is there anything you could do to improve your feelings about keeping food records? _____

_____

_____

Guidelines for Keeping Food Records

Once you have agreed that food records can be a helpful tool in weight management, keep the following guidelines in mind:

1. Buy a small notebook or obtain a checkbook register for keeping your food records. Find something small that you can carry easily with you in your pocket or purse so that it is easy to access. Your record book should have enough room for you to keep track of each day on one sheet. Then, when you are analyzing the records, you won't have to keep flipping pages. The record should have enough pages to keep a week or several weeks in one book. Do not keep track of your records on individual, loose sheets of paper. This method makes it too hard to keep track, and the papers easily get lost. See the blank record sheet in Appendix C. You might like to make copies of it and keep them in a binder.

2. Once you have your food records, write down each food as you eat it. Use your record book to keep track of at least the food and calories you consume. Some people also find it useful to note the people they are with, where they eat, their moods, and any other information that might be pertinent. If you do not know the number of calories in a certain food while you are eating it, look it up as soon as you have access to a calorie book.

3. Learn portion sizes, and write them down. At first, you will need to weigh and measure everything you eat to determine accurately what you are eating. As you become more skilled at this activity, you will know portion sizes just by looking at a food. Even then, it is a good idea to spot-check yourself for accuracy. Always write down the amount you eat., How much you eat is as important as what you eat.

4. Total your calorie intake after each meal or snack so that you know at all times where you stand in your "calorie budget." Doing so allows you to be proactive instead of reactive regarding your food choices. Watching the calories add up every time you eat can be painful, but it also helps you see where you stand.

Box 5 shows a sample food record.

Using Food Records

Now let's play detective. What kind of information can you gather from the food record in Box 5? This person needs about 1,800 calories per day to maintain her weight if she does not exercise. Her calorie goal was 1,400 calories per day. She exceeded that level, and by looking at her records, it's easy to see where she ran into trouble.

For example, she ate a third of her total calorie intake at dinner. She scored herself a 5 for hunger for each meal (on a scale of 1 to 5, with 5 being the most hungry). She said she was lonely at dinner. She ate 775 calories for breakfast and lunch but had very limited amounts of protein. Go back through the food records and look for suspicious behaviors and situations that led to her overeating. Write them below.

_____

_____

_____

_____

_____

_____

Now determine how this information could be used for problem solving. For example, this person was very hungry and lonely at dinner. Maybe if she had an apple on the way home, planned a low-calorie meal, and had a friend over, she would eat a lighter dinner. She also could have eaten a more balanced breakfast and lunch. Maybe then she would not have wanted the snacks in the

BOX 5: SAMPLE FOOD RECORD

Time	Food and Portion Size	Calories	Hunger*	Mood	With	Where	Running Daily Calorie Total
7:00 A.M.	3-ounce bagel	225	5	Stressed	Self	Kitchen table	
	2 teaspoons grape jelly	35					
	Coffee	0					
	2 teaspoons nonfat milk	10					270
8:30 A.M.	Coffee	0	0	Happy	Self	Desk	
	2 teaspoons whole milk	15					285
12:00 P.M.	2 cups garden salad	10	5	Happy	Molly		
	2 tablespoons fat-free ranch salad dressing	30					
	4-ounce bran muffin	400					
	2 cups coffee	0					
	2 individual-sized containers half-and-half	50					775
3:00 P.M.	1 ounce pretzels	100	4	Tired	Self	Desk	
	1-ounce chocolate chip cookie	135					1,010
6:00 P.M.	3-ounce hamburger	225	5	Lonely	Self	Kitchen table	
	2 ounces white bread	150					
	1 tablespoon ketchup	30					
	½ cup potato salad	130					
	3 ounces wine	110					1,655
8:30 P.M.	1 cup sugar-free hot chocolate	50	1	Tired	Self	Couch	
	1-ounce peanut butter cookie	135					1,840

*Scale of 1 to 5, with 5 being the most hungry.

Total daily calories: 1,840
Physical activity: 1 hour aerobics (465 calories)

Calories burned in physical activity (calculated using Table 2): 465 calories
Weekly weight: 6/6: 165 pounds (before breakfast)

afternoon. Use the clues you wrote down in the last exercise and write down solutions here.

_____

_____

_____

What different food choices could she have made that would have kept her calorie intake down? Also, she did not eat any fruit or dairy products (except the milk in her coffee), and not enough from the meat/protein group. What different food choices would have been more nutritious? For example, instead of the bran muffin, she could have had 1 cup of fat-free, sugar-free yogurt (savings: 300 calories). She also could have requested nonfat or low-fat milk for her coffee. Replacing at least one of the cookies

with a piece of fruit would have saved some calories and added some nutrients. Can you find other ways she could have kept her calories down and added some vitamins and minerals?

_____

_____

This exercise should give you an idea as to how you can use your own food records in your own problem solving.

Remember the golden rules of record keeping: Keep the records with you, write down what you eat when you eat it, write down portion sizes, and keep a running total throughout the day.

Move It and Lose It!
—*Physical Activity*

A lot of evidence suggests that one of the key reasons Western nations are experiencing an obesity epidemic is because of "couch potato syndrome" (in Japan, they call it "Nintendo syndrome"). Because of everything from drive-through windows to dishwashers, even children hardly get any activity. Yet research also suggests that regular physical activity is one of the factors most strongly associated with long-term weight-loss success. Unfortunately, many people balk at the thought of exercise. This attitude is due in part to *learned aversions.* People learn to hate working out because, in the past, they started out at full speed—jogging 7 days a week at the highest speed they could maintain and going uphill. With such a starting point, either injury or early burnout is inevitable. But what if walking for just 10 minutes were enough? Would that make the thought of becoming an exerciser more palatable?

In reality, as discussed in the section on goal setting, small, realistic goals are more effective than overwhelming ones. Exercising for 10 minutes 2 or 3 times a week is an excellent way to develop the habit of physical activity. It is hard not to find 10 minutes in even the busiest day to get moving. That is to say, there are no excuses. What good will 10 minutes do? you might ask. Studies have found that three 10-minute bouts of physical activity can have almost the same positive effects on health as a single 30-minute bout. Further, long-term weight loss is a marathon, not a sprint, so to speak. It may not be enough in the long run to be active for only 10 minutes a day; but 10 minutes a day consistently over a lifetime will have a more positive outcome than 2 hours a day for 6 weeks, and then nothing. Further, 10 minutes is a starting place. From 10 minutes, you can build up to 11 minutes and keep on going.

To illustrate, a former athlete gained a large amount of weight upon retiring. His only physical activity was to go to the refrigerator, the bathroom, and bed. His first physical activity goal was to go outside and check the mail, which he did faithfully. Eventually, as he simultaneously lost weight, activity became easier, and he began walking for 10 minutes. He continued and slowly added running to his program. Seeing more and more results from both diet and physical activity inspired him to increase his time commitment to physical activity. Eventually, he progressed from his 5-minute trip to the mailbox to running the vertical mile race in New York City, up the stairs of the Empire State Building.

In addition to having a formal physical activity plan, increasing activities of daily living is another way to burn extra calories. Examples include getting up to change the television channel, parking far away from an entrance, performing more activities by hand instead of using labor-saving devices, and going down the hallway to talk to a coworker instead of using the telephone. Although they may not seem like much, these little activities add up.

List five ways you can increase activity in your life:

1. _____

2. _____

3. _____

4. _____

5. _____

Now list some obstacles to getting started with your physical activity exercise plan (for example, "no time," "hurt my foot," or "tired when I get home"). Write down the obstacle, and then counter it with a possible solution.

Obstacle   *Solution*

_____   _____

_____   _____

_____   _____

_____   _____

_____   _____

Confronting your excuses is a great start!

Types of Physical Activity

We can divide physical activity into three basic categories: *aerobic activity, muscle strength and endurance,* and *flexibility*. Each type of physical activity is important, and each benefits us in different ways.

AEROBIC ACTIVITY

For long-term weight loss and burning calories, aerobic exercise is essential. Both the surgeon general and the American College of Sports Medicine recommend a minimum of 30 minutes per day of moderate physical activity at least 5 days a week for weight management, with 60 minutes being optimal.

So what is aerobic exercise? *Aerobic exercise* is activity that uses the large muscles—such as the quadriceps at the front of the thigh—in a continuous, rhythmic pattern. Examples include dancing fast, bike riding, walking, and swimming. Examples of aerobic activities that meet the surgeon general's recommendation for "moderate physical activity"* include the following:

- Playing basketball (shooting baskets) for 30 minutes.
- Bicycling 5 miles in 30 minutes.
- Dancing fast for 30 minutes.
- Gardening for 30 minutes to 45 minutes.
- Running 1.5 miles in 15 minutes.
- Swimming laps for 20 minutes.
- Walking 2 miles in 30 minutes.
- Washing and waxing a car for 45 minutes to 60 minutes.

- Washing windows or floors for 50 minutes to 60 minutes.
- Wheeling yourself in a wheelchair for 30 minutes to 40 minutes.

Aerobic activity benefits people by burning extra calories and helping to keep weight down, increasing levels of "good cholesterol" in the blood, controlling high blood pressure, keeping bones strong (true for some types of aerobic activity, such as walking or jogging), and increasing the efficiency of the heart.

To be truly effective, however, aerobic activity must meet certain standards. First, it must be performed for at least 30 minutes (although recent evidence suggests that three 10-minute bouts may be effective). Second, the intensity of the aerobic activity must be high enough (as little as 50 percent of your maximum heart rate range may be enough to promote improvement). Third, you must undertake aerobic activity at least 3 days a week.

To determine your maximum heart rate (beats per minute), subtract your age from 220. Then divide by 2 to determine a good starting level:

$$\frac{220 - age}{2}$$

For example, if you are 40 years old,

$$220 - 40 = 180$$
$$180 \div 2 = 90$$

Thus, your heart rate goal initially should be 90 beats per minute. To measure your heart rate,

*Source: National Heart, Lung, and Blood Institute. Guide to physical activity. Available at: http://www.nhlbi.nih.gov/health/public/heart/obesity/lose_wt/phy_act.htm. Accessed April 26, 2003.

PAR-Q & YOU

(A Questionnaire for People Aged 15 to 69)

Regular physical activity is fun and healthy, and increasingly more people are starting to become more active every day. Being more active is very safe for most people. However, some people should check with their doctor before they start becoming much more physically active.

If you are planning to become much more physically active than you are now, start by answering the seven questions in the box below. If you are between the ages of 15 and 69, the PAR-Q will tell you if you should check with your doctor before you start. If you are over 69 years of age, and you are not used to being very active, check with your doctor.

Common sense is your best guide when you answer these questions. Please read the questions carefully and answer each one honestly: check YES or NO.

YES	NO	
☐	☐	**1. Has your doctor ever said that you have a heart condition <u>and</u> that you should only do physical activity recommended by a doctor?**
☐	☐	**2. Do you feel pain in your chest when you do physical activity?**
☐	☐	**3. In the past month, have you had chest pain when you were not doing physical activity?**
☐	☐	**4. Do you lose your balance because of dizziness or do you ever lose consciousness?**
☐	☐	**5. Do you have a bone or joint problem (for example, back, knee or hip) that could be made worse by a change in your physical activity?**
☐	☐	**6. Is your doctor currently prescribing drugs (for example, water pills) for your blood pressure or heart condition?**
☐	☐	**7. Do you know of <u>any other reason</u> why you should not do physical activity?**

If you answered

YES to one or more questions.

Talk with your doctor by phone or in person BEFORE you start becoming much more physically active or BEFORE you have a fitness appraisal. Tell your doctor about the PAR-Q and which questions you answered YES.

- You may be able to do any activity you want — as long as you start slowly and build up gradually. Or, you may need to restrict your activities to those which are safe for you. Talk with your doctor about the kinds of activities you wish to participate in and follow his/her advice.
- Find out which community programs are safe and helpful for you.

NO to all questions.

If you answered NO honestly to <u>all</u> PAR-Q questions, you can be reasonably sure that you can:
- start becoming much more physically active — begin slowly and build up gradually. This is the safest and easiest way to go.
- take part in a fitness appraisal — this is an excellent way to determine your basic fitness so that you can plan the best way for you to live actively. It is also highly recommended that you have your blood pressure evaluated. If your reading is over 144/94, talk with your doctor before you start becoming much more physically active.

→ DELAY BECOMING MUCH MORE ACTIVE:
- if you are not feeling well because of a temporary illness such as a cold or a fever — wait until you feel better; or
- if you are or may be pregnant — talk to your doctor before you start becoming more active.

PLEASE NOTE: If your health changes so that you then answer YES to any of the above questions, tell your fitness or health professional. Ask whether you should change your physical activity plan.

<u>Informed Use of the PAR-Q</u>: The Canadian Society for Exercise Physiology, Health Canada, and their agents assume no liability for persons who undertake physical activity, and if in doubt after completing this questionnaire, consult your doctor prior to physical activity.

No changes permitted. You are encouraged to photocopy the PAR-Q but only if you use the entire form.

NOTE: If the PAR-Q is being given to a person before he or she participates in a physical activity program or a fitness appraisal, this section may be used for legal or administrative purposes.

"I have read, understood and completed this questionnaire. Any questions I had were answered to my full satisfaction."

NAME _____

SIGNATURE _____ DATE_____

SIGNATURE OF PARENT _____ WITNESS _____
or GUARDIAN (for participants under the age of majority)

Note: This physical activity clearance is valid for a maximum of 12 months from the date it is completed and becomes invalid if your condition changes so that you would answer YES to any of the seven questions.

 © Canadian Society for Exercise Physiology   Supported by: Health   Santé
Canada   Canada

Figure 3: PAR-Q and You. *Source:* Physical Activity Readiness Questionnaire (PAR-Q) © 2002. Reprinted with permission from the Canadian Society for Exercise Physiology. http://www.csep.ca/forms.asp

place your right index and middle fingers lightly over your right carotid artery (the artery by your Adam's apple). You can find this spot by placing your middle finger above your index finger on your Adam's apple and then sliding them to the right until you reach the groove in your neck, at which point you should be able to feel your pulse. Measure it for 10 seconds, and multiply this number by 6. This number is your heart rate.

As your fitness level improves, you may want to increase the *intensity* of your activity to 60 percent or 70 percent of your maximum heart rate range. To determine this level, follow the formula you just used; instead of dividing by 2, though, multiply by 0.6 (for 60 percent) or 0.7 (for 70 percent). In any case, you should be able to carry on a conversation comfortably while exercising. If you cannot, you are probably working too hard.

You must undertake aerobic activity at least 3 days a week. (The American College of Sports Medicine recommends 5 days a week for weight control, and the *Surgeon General's Report on Physical Activity* recommends daily activity as optimal.)

Exercise also should be preceded by 5 minutes of warming up (slow walking, for example) and be followed by 5 minutes of cooling down to prevent injury. Stretching before and after is also crucial. **NOTE**: *During physical activity, if you feel any chest pain, dizziness, light-headedness, extreme shortness of breath, muscle or skeletal pain, or extreme fatigue, stop exercising immediately.*

Before beginning a physical activity program, answer the questions in Figure 3, and obtain a clearance from your doctor as indicated. If you are over 69 years of age and sedentary, check with your doctor.

MUSCLE STRENGTH AND ENDURANCE

Aerobic activity will tone the muscles used for that activity. Leg muscles will become stronger and firmer with walking, and arm and leg muscles will become stronger and firmer with swimming. However, you must perform resistance exercises to tone muscles in other parts of the body. Resistance exercises include weight training, pulling elastic bands, calisthenics, and similar types of exercises. Using heavier weights or greater resistance with fewer repetitions will serve to develop larger muscles, whereas using lighter weights or lower resistance with more repetitions will tone and improve muscle endurance rather than build muscle. Although these exercises build and/or tone muscles, they will not get rid of fat in specific areas, such as the stomach. Only overall fat loss can do that.

FLEXIBILITY

Flexibility, the third type of physical activity, has become more popular in recent years. Yoga is an example of a flexibility physical activity that is offered through many gyms and community centers. Increased flexibility reduces the risk of injury and increases the range of motion of a muscle (meaning that you can stretch it farther).

For assistance in setting up and starting a safe and effective physical activity program for yourself, seek professional assistance through a certified personal trainer or exercise physiologist or through a licensed physical therapist. Reputable organizations include the American College of Sports Medicine and the American Council on Exercise.

Sticking with It

Like thousands of others, you probably started an exercise program in the past, and you've probably also dropped that program. If so, you already may have addressed the obstacles and possible solutions. Remember, an exercise or physical activity program is a marathon, not a sprint. What you do over the long haul is far more important than what you do for the next month if you don't keep it up. Here are some tried-and-true steps for successfully starting and maintaining a workout regimen:

1. Use the buddy system. Find an activity partner who is committed to starting and sticking with a regular physical activity program. Make sure that you don't support each other's excuses, though!

2.   Try to cater your physical activity program to your needs. If you hate exercising indoors, then a gym probably won't be the solution for you. If you have bad knees, running may be out of the question.

3.   Set specific, realistic goals. Make sure they are goals you are likely to achieve.

4.   Be realistic. You will not be able to lose 20 pounds in a month. Your waist will not go from 40 inches to 25 inches in 2 months. Aiming for the impossible will get you discouraged and frustrated, even though your progress may be tremendous in human terms.

5.   Write up a contract stating your plan, and sign it with one of your supporters.

6.   Establish a nonfood reward system for yourself upon completion of the small goals you have set.

7.   Use a pedometer. A pedometer is a great way to track your activity, reinforce and encourage activity, and facilitate goal setting.

8.   Obtain measurements at regular time intervals, such as each month. Measurements are preferable to weight to chart your progress, because you may gain muscle weight while losing inches. You may even contact a local gym to see if it determines body-fat measurements. These measurements provide objective information about the good results of your program. Positive changes in measurements are generally very motivating and rewarding in themselves.

Now take a moment to think about and write down the types of activities you have enjoyed in the past:

_____

_____

_____

_____

What would you like to establish as a long-term (say, 1-year) physical activity goal? Break that goal down into smaller goals—6-month, 3-month, 1-month, and 1-week goals:

One year from now, I would like to _____.

Six months from now, I would like to _____.

Three months from now, I would like to _____.

One month from now, I would like to _____.

To start working toward my goals, this week I will _____

_____.

Cyber Support

The National Weight Control Registry maintains a Web site with inspirational success stories of how others lost weight and kept it off. You also can read some of the latest research findings there and find links to other useful weight-control Web sites. After becoming a success story yourself, you can register and share your strategies. The Web site's address is http://www.lifespan.org/services/bmed/wt_loss/nwcr/.

"The Devil Made Me Do It!"
—Reducing Temptation

Many people think that losing weight is simply a matter of willpower. When it comes to willpower, it seems, some people have it, and some people don't. People who have it are strong, and they are lucky. People who don't have willpower are just plain out of luck. Some dieters say things like "I should be able to keep cake in the house for my family and not eat it. Why should my family have to suffer just because I am weak?" Others say, "I should be able to go to a buffet without breaking my diet." What are some of the ways you rely on willpower alone because of the "shoulds" you tell yourself?

People tend to assume that individuals who are thin can simply resist temptation, just don't like high-calorie foods, or were born thin and don't have to worry about their weight. However, it is not that simple. Some people are successful because they apply more skills to weight loss. There are many skills you can apply to increase your chances of success.

Many people are successful at maintaining a desirable weight by setting themselves up for success and avoiding temptation. For example, Pat was a great cook and had always had the family over for dinner on special occasions. But one year Pat was trying to lose weight, and she had been quite successful to date. She was a little bit nervous about her grandchild's birthday party, which she was hosting the next week. Pat planned for success during this event in several ways. First, she thought about things in advance. She knew she had a history of overeating and that to break this pattern, she would have to do some things differently. Second, Pat made a commitment to stay within her dietary guidelines during this

event. Finally, Pat came up with a plan: She would prepare a main dish that she didn't like but that the family really liked—in this case, a beef roast. Then she decided to cook plenty of vegetables (low fat) so that there would be things that she could eat. She also decided that she would bake a cake that wasn't a big favorite of hers. So she wouldn't feel deprived, she got herself a treat that would fit into her diet plan. Later, she sent all of the leftovers home with her children so the food wouldn't be around to tempt her. She also lost a pound that week. You see, Pat planned in advance ways to limit the temptation, and she set herself up for success.

Here are some other ways to limit temptation:

- ■ Don't keep leftovers in clear containers.
- ■ Ask the people you live with to hide tempting snacks.
- ■ If you have decided to eat a high-calorie food, buy single-serving containers.
- ■ Don't look at the snack machines at work.
- ■ Don't go down the cookie, snack, or bakery aisles at the grocery store.

Write down some other ways you can reduce the temptations in your life:

_____

_____

_____

_____

Losing weight is very difficult. Why make it any harder on yourself than it has to be? Anything you can do to reduce temptation increases your chances of success.

Gaining Support

Trying to lose weight without support is like trying to swim upstream. Many research studies have shown that people who have good support are more successful at weight loss and weight maintenance. Support can come in a variety of forms and from a variety of sources. It can be as simple as being congratulated on your recent weight loss or acknowledged for sticking to your commitment during a tough time. It can also be more involved. For instance, for you to feel totally supported, perhaps your spouse will need to stop bringing home fresh-cooked doughnuts in the morning or agree to keep high-calorie foods in the garage.

Some people have a hard time getting the support they need at home. Luckily, outside sources of support are also available. For example, weight-loss groups or counselors can serve as support systems. Good friends are another source of support. Think about some people or resources you can look to for support. Sometimes people have sources of support but fail to let them know their support is needed or what that support might be. Because support is so important in weight-loss success and may be difficult to obtain, try the following exercises to explore this issue.

Support Exercises

Some people have a hard time sharing their needs with others. Perhaps they are afraid of criticism. Maybe they do not feel they deserve support. Have you ever needed or wanted someone's help with your weight loss but did not let that person know? If so, take a few minutes to explore that situation. What were some of the feelings you had about asking the person for help?

_____

_____

_____

How can you overcome some of those feelings about asking for help? The next exercise will help you challenge your feelings. Keep in mind

that you do not necessarily have to agree with what you write. You just have to start by recognizing the possibilities.

Let's say that you determined that you did not ask your friend for support at the last party you went to because you thought she would think you were weak. When you thought about it further, you realized that *you* were the one who thought you were weak. Upon realizing this fact, you can challenge that thought by stating that asking for support is not a sign of weakness—that everyone can benefit from support. Use this statement as an affirmation to change your ideas about asking for support. Read this affirmation every night and several times a day. Gradually, you may find that you actually start to believe it yourself. Now take a few minutes to "challenge" the feelings you outlined before:

_____

_____

_____

Next, think about some behaviors that your family, friends, coworkers, and others engage in that do not support your weight-loss efforts. An example might be the following: "When my friends and I get together, they always want to go to the pizza place that doesn't have a salad bar. I enjoy the friendship, so I want to go, but when we get there and there isn't anything I can eat, I cave in and eat pizza." Write an example from your own experience:

_____

_____

_____

_____

Now think about some ways in which your friends, family, coworkers, or others can support you (for example, "It would be helpful to me if my friends would agree to dine out at places that offer low-calorie foods"):

_____

_____

_____

_____

_____

Communicating Your Needs

Once you have determined how friends and family can offer you support and you have become open to asking for that support, you need to communicate your needs to others. This step is hard for many people, so here are some pointers:

1. Use "I" statements. Do not say things that blame other people for your problems. Simply let them know how they can help you. By doing so, you will avoid putting others on the defensive. For instance, it sounds a lot different to say "I can't stay on my diet because you keep eating fattening foods in front of me" than to say "I have a difficult time resisting fattening foods when they are around me." The first statement blames the other person for your inability to stick with your eating plan. It can stimulate a defensive response. In the second statement, you have owned the fact that you have a hard time resisting food when there are fattening foods around, and no one can argue with you. This consequence is good, because arguing is not your goal. Your goal is to win the help of others. Now, use an "I" statement to let someone know how he or she is not helpful to you:

   _____

   _____

2. Let others know how they can be more helpful to you. If you had the problem described in point number 1, you might say, "It would be helpful to me if you would avoid eating fattening foods in front of me, either by eating them before you come home or by letting me know so that I can leave the room." Write down a

statement to let another person know how he or she can help you solve the problem you described while reading about the first pointer:

_____

_____

_____

3. Do not assume that people should be able to read your mind and intuitively know how to help you. If you are having a problem with another person, you must let that person know.

4. Do not assume that telling someone something one time is adequate. Remember that this is your problem, that it is more important to you, and that you are more likely to remember the issue. The other person may sincerely want to help but may need to be reminded—perhaps more than once. If you have honestly tried to solicit help but feel that you are not getting anywhere, you may need to bring this problem up for discussion. Doing so can be hard, especially if you do not think you are worth the support or believe you "should" be able to lose weight on your own. Remember your earlier exploration of some of the ideas and beliefs that make it hard to ask for help? You may need to practice some self-talk that challenges these beliefs. This step of challenging your destructive self-talk will be an important one for you in overcoming these beliefs.

5. If you have tried and are not able to get the support you need from the people around you, an outside support group may be your best option. You can seek help from reputable weight-loss groups such as Weight Watchers, TOPS, and Overeaters Anonymous, as well as individual counselors and registered dietitians.

6. Even if you have a great support base, weight loss is still ultimately up to you, and solving problems remains your responsibility.

EXERCISE

Find a person with whom you feel safe. It can be a friend, significant other, therapist, or anyone else. Just be sure the person is supportive. Ask the individual to role-play a scenario with you and to take the part of a person who tends to push food on you or otherwise cause you distress in relation to your weight-loss goals. While the person plays the role of the troublesome individual who pushes food on you (for example), assert yourself using the tools you have learned so far. It may be helpful to write down what you will say to this person, though you do not have to use what you have written. Actually going through the motions

of the desired behavior can be a powerful tool in helping you in real situations. A highly recommended book to assist you in developing assertive behaviors is *Your Perfect Right: Assertiveness and Equality in Your Life and Relationships*, 8th edition, by Robert E. Alberti and Michael L. Emmons (Atascadero, Calif: Impact Publishers, 2001).

Some people say that losing weight is the hardest thing they ever tried to do. Having support can go a long way toward successful weight management. Practicing some techniques for obtaining support may give you the extra boost you need.

Have Faith . . .
in Yourself

In the 1970s, a psychologist performed an experiment that suggested a phenomenon called *learned helplessness*. In his experiment, he put some dogs in a cage to which an electrical shock could be applied. One group of dogs had a way to escape the shock, and they quickly learned that if they jumped over a wall, they would be fine. The other group of dogs did not have a way to escape and had to endure the shock. What this researcher found, though, was that when he later provided these dogs with a way to escape, they still just sat there and endured the shock. From this finding he concluded that the dogs had learned that no matter what they did, they could not escape, and so they did nothing. He termed this behavior *learned helplessness.*

The same type of behavior may occur in dieters who have set themselves up for failure in the past. People who have followed diets with claims such as "Lose 10 pounds in a week," "Eat all you want and still lose weight," or "Lose weight by eating only bananas and hot dogs" have been misled. The bananas-and-hot-dogs diet claims you can "follow this diet, and you are guar-

anteed to lose." Then, after 2 weeks of eating nothing but bananas and hot dogs, you "cheat." What the claims don't tell you is that it takes the will of Hercules to stay with such a diet for any length of time. However, when you go off the diet, you believe that you are the problem. In reality, it is often the diet, goal, or process that is the problem.

Many posters, books, and public speakers tell you that you must believe in yourself to achieve your goals. Sometimes dieters must overcome past defeats and move forward with confidence. This is easier said than done, though. A couple of behaviors that can help are setting realistic goals to increase your self-confidence and practicing self-affirmation, or positive self-talk. Many of the beliefs people have about themselves are based on things that they and others have said to and about them. If people hear a message often enough, they start to believe it. If the message is a positive one about themselves, they develop a positive self-image. If the message is negative, they develop a negative self-image. Think about the analogy of two hungry dogs, one mean and one nice. If you feed the mean dog, he just grows and grows while the nice dog gets weaker. If, in contrast, you feed the nice dog, he gets stronger and stronger while the mean dog gets weaker. Self-affirmations serve the same purpose. If you can feed your self-image positive messages, your positive self-image gets stronger. By the same token, if you can ignore, or "starve," the negative messages, they will get weaker. You may not even believe a positive message at first, but feed the positive image anyway. Eventually, as it becomes stronger, you will begin to believe your self-affirmation.

What are some self-defeating things that you say to yourself regarding your weight and your ability to lose weight?

_____

_____

_____

_____

_____

What are some affirmations you can tell yourself to overcome your self-defeating self-talk?

_____

_____

_____

_____

_____

_____

Write these positive statements down, and post them in a few places, just as you did with your goals. They will remind you to repeat these affirmations to yourself. And when you catch yourself making negative comments to yourself about your ability to lose weight or about your self-worth, challenge those thoughts with positive thoughts. Even if you don't believe them at first, follow the process. Eventually you will begin to believe the positive thoughts.

When Size Matters
—Portion Control

Portion size is often the missing link in weight management. Many dieters and calorie books calculate the calories in various food items based on "a piece" or "a serving." The listing in one popular calorie book for a muffin is 180 calories. That amount may be accurate if the muffin weighs about 2 ounces and does not have nuts. But what if it is a 6-ounce muffin with nuts? This muffin would probably check in at about 600 calories—a difference of 420 calories. Assuming that your goal is to lose 1 pound a week by eating 500 fewer calories per day, this one error made every day will cost you your 1-pound weight loss. No wonder you're on a plateau!

Portion size is a vitally important component of weight loss and management. When you make the commitment to weight loss, you will have to weigh and measure everything until you have an idea of what various serving sizes look like. After a couple of weeks, though, you will start to recognize portion sizes and may not need to be as rigid. However, it is a good idea to spot-check yourself every now and then to be sure your portion sizes haven't started creeping up.

To learn portion sizes, you will need to have a set of dry-measuring cups, measuring spoons, a liquid-measuring cup, and a good food scale. Once you have this equipment, you can simplify things a bit by, say, measuring how much a certain ladle or bowl holds. Then you'll know that whenever you eat a bowl of cereal, you are eating a certain amount. You must still be careful to avoid "heaping" servings. Using such servings is a way dieters can lie to themselves and cheat without really having to confront it (although it still shows up on the scales).

Here's another hint to use if you have access to a 4-cup glass measuring cup. Fill this measuring cup with enough water that when you put your hand in it, the water will go up to your wrist without going past the 4-cup mark. Note the measurement before you stick your hand in; then dunk your hand in the water up to your wrist. While your hand is in the water, note the measurement. Subtract the reading taken when your hand is out of the water from the reading with your hand in the water to learn how big your fist is. For example, say the water level in the measuring cup was 2 cups without your hand and 3 cups with your hand; 3 cups minus 2 cups equals 1 cup, so your fist is about 1 cup. Now you can use your fist as a com-

BOX 6: COMMON MEASURES

3 teaspoons = 1 tablespoon
16 tablespoons = 1 cup
16 ounces = 1 pound
1 tablespoon (liquid) = ½ ounce
1 cup (liquid) = 8 ounces
1 ounce = 28 grams
1 cup (liquid) = 240 milliliters

parison to estimate portion sizes when you do not have access to measuring cups and food scales. Some other important information about determining portion sizes is listed in Box 6.

No-Calorie Treats

Food is a very convenient item people use to take care of themselves. It tastes good and is pleasant. It is easily available (too available, some would say). It is affordable. It is also something that many people have been conditioned since childhood to use as a treat or reward. Food can be a form of rebellion or a way to have some control over life. If you are trying to lose weight, it may be helpful to break the pattern of using food as a reward or treat. But to set yourself up for success, you might consider first establishing a list of no-calorie treats that you can use instead of food. Some ideas for rewards that successful dieters have developed in the past include the following:

- Buying fresh flowers.
- Calling a good friend on the telephone.
- Enjoying music.
- Taking 10 minutes just to do nothing.
- Going to a nice coffee shop to have some gourmet coffee or tea.
- Putting on a relaxation CD that takes you to a nice place.
- Making a list of ten things for which you are truly grateful.

- Setting aside a small amount of money each time you accomplish one of your goals. (When you feel you need a treat or reward, use this money for that purpose. Perhaps you can have your nails done, buy a book, or get a massage.)

What are some ideas for taking care of yourself without food?

_____

_____

_____

_____

_____

Refer to this list when you catch yourself looking for food as a reward.

Another way in which nonfood rewards can be useful is in providing incentives for achieving goals. Although many people say that losing weight is enough of a reward in itself, it is still helpful to give yourself an external treat as an official pat on the back. When you have a hard time getting started, setting up a reward system for sticking with your calorie plan, keeping records, exercising, or reaching other goals can help. Decide what incentive would help you stay with your program. It can be anything that is desirable to you. Some examples include setting aside time to read a book you enjoy or buying a shirt that you want. Whatever it is, it should be something that you give yourself *if and only if* you achieve the goal you decided on. It cannot be something that you would give yourself anyway. Also, you can't decide afterward that you really don't deserve the reward after all and then not give it to yourself. If you have achieved your goal, you deserve the reward. That's part of the deal. Don't let yourself down.

If you are having a really hard time losing weight or finding a powerful reward, here is an idea that works well: money. Money is one of the most powerful incentives available, and it is universally popular. Of course, the idea of giving it up is not popular, and that's why it works. In one study, a group of subjects agreed that they would write a check to their favorite charity each week. They gave the check for 5 dollars to the

researcher. If they lost weight that week, they got the check back. If they didn't lose weight, they didn't get the check back. Another group did not participate in the reward system. Week after week, the group that wrote the checks lost more weight than the group that did not. There was one problem, though: Not many people were willing to participate. But you can see that for the ones who did, the results were great. So if you want to get serious about losing weight, consider setting up such an agreement. Maybe a spouse, relative, or friend will work with you to help you stay honest and withhold or reimburse your checks.

This week, set up a reward system. Ask yourself these questions:

- What is the goal you want to achieve?
- What is the reward you will give yourself if you meet your goal?

Write down the answers; then give yourself the reward when you reach your goal.

"Chain, Chain, Chain"
—Breaking Your Behavior Chains

When people tackle a problem behavior, they often look only at the undesired end point. Really, though, each behavior is a series of behaviors linked together—similar to the links in a chain. Have you ever heard the expression "A chain is only as strong as its weakest link"? This idea applies to chains of behaviors, too. Therefore, eating behavior can be seen as a chain. In other words, each eating event is a series of behaviors that are linked together like links in a chain. Using this idea, you can take any behavior, such as eating ice cream at night, and break it down from start to finish. Breaking down a behavior into its "links" will allow you to examine it, step by step, for the weakest link. This activity will help you find exactly where in the behavior you are most likely to break the chain.

For example, say that every night on your way home from work you automatically turn into the ice cream shop and buy an ice cream sundae. You have decided that this activity is a problem, because you know that the sundae has 500 calories, and you have not been able to lose even a pound a week. You have decided several times that you would not stop that day, but every day at 5:10, there you are—ordering a sundae. If you break this behavior down into steps, you'll find that it is not one behavior, but a series of behaviors. The sequence is as follows: You get off work. You drive down Food Boulevard. You see Ice Cream Iggy's. You think about ice cream. Your mouth waters. You pull into the parking lot. You stop the car. You go inside. You order a sundae. You pay for the sundae. You take the sundae, and you eat it. You cry and feel discouraged with yourself.

Each step in this process can be altered in some way, any of which may be the "missing link" in solving your behavior problem. Let's examine how you could make some changes in the process:

1. You get off work. You'll still get off work, but perhaps you can act here by getting a diet soda for the trip home.

2. You drive down Food Boulevard. Can you drive down a different street—one that doesn't have as many food joints?

3. You see Ice Cream Iggy's. Can you keep your eyes on the road and not look around as much?

4. You think about ice cream. When you start to think of ice cream, can you divert your thoughts to winning the lottery?

5. Your mouth waters. If you don't see or think about ice cream, you won't have this problem.

6. You pull into the parking lot. Can you stay in the inner lane so that it is not as easy to turn into Ice Cream Iggy's?

7. You stop the car. Can you agree to let the car idle for 5 minutes before you go in so you'll have a little cooling-off time?

8. You go inside. Can you commit to walking around the building first (and thus have *more* cooling-off time)?

9. You order a sundae. Is there anything with fewer calories that you can order?

10. You pay for the sundae. Carry only enough money for a telephone call, and no more. Then you can't buy a sundae!

11. You take the sundae, and you eat it. Can you save some calories from that day's allotment so you can afford the sundae? Can you ask Iggy's to use less ice cream, sauce, and nuts?

 Do you get the idea? Now identify a behavior that is interfering with your weight-loss goals, and break it into individual steps and solutions:

Problem behavior:

_____

_____

Step 1: _____

Solution: _____

Step 2: _____

Solution: _____

Step 3: _____

Solution: _____

Step 4: _____

Solution: _____

Step 5: _____

Solution: _____

Step 6: _____

Solution: _____

Pasta or Prozac?
—Emotions and Eating

When people are feeling sad, angry, stressed, discouraged, or any of a variety of other emotions, the thing they want most is to feel better. If they're angry, feeling better might require that they confront someone. If they're stressed, they might have to prioritize their tasks. If they're sad, they might have to address issues concerning their relationships. In many cases, the solutions may not be very obvious. Even if they are, people may be afraid to practice new skills or may find that these skills take some effort.

One thing that people know will make them feel better is eating. Eating can give a reliable and immediate feeling of relief. Food is easy. It's enjoyable. It's available. It's fast. In many ways, it's the perfect emotional escape. Some people describe food as a friend—the only reliable friend they have. Is it any wonder it is so hard to give it up?

One important concept to remember is that it is easier to replace something with something than to replace it with nothing. Removing food as your friend and therapist can leave you with an empty feeling. If this empty feeling is allowed to grow, as during a time of emotional distress, you are more likely to give in and eat something you shouldn't or to binge. The key is to recognize what role food serves in easing uncomfortable feelings and to find an alternative.

Food and Emotions Exercise

For each of the emotions listed below, think of how food has served you. (For example, for anger you might write, "When I am angry at my mother, I eat. I think I do this because I know she hates that I am overweight. She always has things to say about it!")

Anger: _____
_____
_____
_____

Sadness:_____
_____
_____
_____

Happiness: _____
_____
_____
_____

Fear: _____
_____
_____
_____

Anxiety:_____

_____

_____

_____

Loneliness: _____

_____

_____

_____

Disappointment: _____

_____

_____

_____

Guilt and shame: _____

_____

_____

_____

Hurt: _____

_____

_____

_____

If there are other feelings that you deal with by eating, write them on a separate sheet, and state how you use food to cope with them.

Effective Ways of Dealing with Feelings

Were you able to identify some ways you use food to cope with feelings? In the next exercise, you will identify other, more effective ways to deal with those feelings. For example, John realized that he ate when he was feeling stressed as a way of procrastinating. When he had to deal with an overwhelming or unpleasant task, he would eat instead (it's awfully hard to write a manuscript with a french fry). When he realized this pattern, he also realized that he had some issues he had to address with himself first. Just being aware helped somewhat. But he also had to learn how to avoid procrastinating when faced with unpleasant tasks. John came up with some ideas about how to stop procrastinating by eating food. His ideas included doing his least favorite task first to get it out of the way; rewarding himself with

something noncaloric when he finished the task; and breaking the task into small, manageable pieces. These activities, he thought, would be more direct ways of dealing with his procrastination that would reduce his stress and his calorie intake.

Sometimes you may be aware of a solution but feel overwhelmed by it. Remember that when you come up with a solution, you can break it into small steps and set progressive goals, just as you did for your weight-loss goal. For example, if your goal is to deal with your loneliness, one of your ideas might be signing up for volunteer work. If doing so is intimidating to you, write down the steps you must take. First you must find out what agencies you'd be interested in helping out. Then you must find their telephone numbers. Next you have to call them. You can go from there.

Recognize that many of your feelings are the result of your thinking. Examine what you are telling yourself when you feel bad. Do you have unrealistic expectations of others? Do you expect them to read your mind? Do you expect yourself to be perfect? Do you expect life to be perfect?

Let's look at another example. Ann had been sticking to her diet and exercise plan to the letter. When some out-of-town guests stayed with her for a few days, she developed a plan for staying on track while they visited. However, once they got to her house, she felt so happy and lighthearted that she thought, "Well, I'll just splurge a little while they're here. Then I'll get back to my diet and exercise plan after they leave." Ann's guests have been gone for 3 weeks now, and she still isn't back on track. Even though she is exercising again, she has had a hard time with the diet. She tells herself that she is stupid for having gone off it in the first place and that this round will end up like all past weight-loss efforts. She is depressed and feels like a failure. Because she is depressed, she has been eating more. Because she has lost faith in herself, she is not trying as hard.

The reason for these feelings is that she is beating up on herself. However, the thoughts she has regarding her difficult time dieting are not valid. First of all, the decision to splurge while guests visited was not stupid. Maybe she didn't realize how hard it would be to get back to her diet plan, but that does not mean she is stupid. Second, just because she has had a rough 3 weeks does not mean that she will not succeed. It just means she has had a rough 3 weeks.

The next time you catch yourself feeling depressed and discouraged with yourself, try to look at the things you are saying to yourself. Are they valid, or are you indulging in self-loathing self-talk? Make it a practice to refute these messages. Replace them with productive, nonjudgmental messages. Ann could recognize that her negative self-talk is not productive or realistic. She could reassess the situation and develop constructive solutions. Other general ideas for dealing with feelings include keeping a journal, talking about your feelings into a cassette recorder, talking with trusted others, taking a walk, and listening to relaxation CDs.

Now write down some ways in which you can deal with the feelings that you try to escape through eating. First, write down the feeling; then write down at least one solution. When you find a solution that appeals to you, break it into small steps, if you need to.

_____

_____

_____

_____

_____

_____

_____

_____

_____

_____

_____

_____

_____

_____

Seeking Help

Using food to cope with feelings is ineffective. It is an escape from the problem. The best way to deal with a problem is to face it, not to hide from it. This approach can be very threatening, but it is a very important part of growing. Some people may want to seek help from a counselor or psychologist when they reach this point. If you think that you may be able to go through the process of dealing with feelings rather than escaping, resources are available. You may ask someone you know who has been in counseling for suggestions. You can ask your physician for references. You also can call your community mental health agency. These agencies often provide services on a sliding scale of fees. Universities with graduate-level counseling programs often provide counseling at reduced rates. Many insurance companies help pay for counseling services. You also might find help through self-help groups, such as Overeaters Anonymous. Although taking such a step can be very frightening, it could be the first step in changing your life.

'Tis the Season
—*Special Situations*

Close your eyes and imagine this: You are going along with your weight-management program and doing quite well. You are 20 pounds lighter—the lightest you have been in years. You are on a long-awaited trip to the islands, for which you have bought a new wardrobe. What do you look like? How do you feel? What will you be doing on your vacation? What does it feel like to be wearing these clothes? Are you able to do activities that you couldn't do before? What are your meal choices? What are your snack choices? Mentally go through this process, picturing every detail.

Now compare this scene to vacation scenes of the past. What were you wearing? What did you look like? What activities did you participate in? How did you feel about yourself? Were you out on the beach, or were you hiding in the shops?

You probably noticed a difference between vacations past and vacations present or yet to come. Vacations and holidays are times when people want to let down their guard, relax, and have fun. But statistics point out that there is a price for all this fun. The average person gains 7 pounds between Thanksgiving and New Year's Day. And that's an average, meaning that some people gain more than that. As for fun in the sun, many people bring back tales of 10- or 15-pound weight gains from their vacations.

However, there are also tales of success stories during vacations and holidays. For example, Carlos went on a Caribbean cruise while trying to lose weight and improve his health. Cruises are well known for having delicious food available in abundance at several times of the day and night—foods that are loaded with rich sauces and made with cream, butter, fatty meats, and cheese. Such a spread would be hard to resist. But Carlos made plans in advance of his trip. He telephoned the travel agent and let him know that he had certain dietary needs, which the chef on the cruise willingly accommodated. When he returned from the cruise, Carlos reported having had a great time (in spite of the low-calorie food), and he did not gain any weight—a remarkable feat for anyone!

Similar stories can be told about holiday successes. One key to success includes establishing a game plan. Think about how Carlos made plans in advance to be sure that some low-calorie foods would be available for him. For the holidays, if you know you have a lot of holiday parties to attend, you can develop strategies to reduce temptation. If you go to a potluck dinner, for example, bring a low-calorie specialty so that you'll have at least one healthy choice available to you. When neighbors and friends bring you cookies, try one cookie each of your two favorites, and then get them out of the house (even if it means throwing them out or giving them away).

At holiday meals, fill your plate with the low-calorie foods (assuming there are some), and leave room for only one bite of each of the other foods. Make a commitment out loud to have only one plate of food. If you do this, you may be too embarrassed to get seconds (which you know you don't need anyhow). And before you attend a high-calorie affair or vacation, sit down and determine your goals (for example, to maintain your weight and not make food the center of the party or vacation, but to enjoy other activities). Think about how you will accomplish your goals. Mentally go through the event, picturing yourself as a success. Identify the behaviors you are engaging in that will make you successful. Decide what your commitment to yourself will be. Put this commitment in writing so that you will have it with you as a reminder. Finally, remember that holidays and vacations are special times that are meant to be enjoyed, but that there is no excuse for overindulging.

 Write down some specific strategies you can use during special occasions to help you achieve your weight goal. Do not stop until you come up with twenty ideas:

1. _____
2. _____
3. _____
4. _____
5. _____
6. _____
7. _____
8. _____
9. _____
10. _____
11. _____
12. _____
13. _____
14. _____
15. _____
16. _____
17. _____
18. _____
19. _____
20. _____

First Things First
—Setting Priorities

So much to do; so little time! So many competing demands! It's easy to let your weight-loss commitment fall into the background. There will be days when exercising just doesn't seem to fit in. There will be days when you just don't want to fight with the kids, so you buy the snack cakes they want. Or maybe you sometimes think that you just can't be bothered to weigh and measure portion sizes. You may wonder if you really need to plan your meals a week in advance. Isn't there an easier way? Do you sometimes feel that it takes too much emotional energy to continue to ask your family to support you, or to send a wrong order back to the kitchen?

But you must ask for support, and you must send back a wrong order! These everyday, little decisions add up to weight-loss success. Yes, losing weight takes work. No, it never lets up. If you want to lose weight and keep it off, the decisions you make on a day-to-day, minute-to-minute basis are the decisions that determine your success or failure. Lots of things are tugging at you, trying to grab your attention. But diet, physical activity, and factors that influence them must receive priority.

What does it mean for weight loss to receive priority? It means that sometimes you will let people down (which is most difficult for people who live to please others). For example, you may have to tell the kids, "No peanut butter chocolate bars in the house until I feel stronger," or tell your spouse, "None of my famous authentic New York cheesecake until after I lose weight." They may beg. They may plead. They may whine. They may say things like "If you loved me. . . ." But you must stick to your guns. Tell them, "No! I can't.

At least not for now." Then turn it back on them. Let them know how important their support is to you. Tell them that if they loved *you*. . . .

When weight loss receives priority, it also means no more excuses. It may seem that there is no good day for exercise, no easy time to pass up a candy bar, and no easy way to become assertive or more outgoing. True, at times these things will be more difficult, but commitment insists that you move onward, through the fog, thin-ly and fit-ly.

Now it's time for self-exploration. Think about which people, events, and circumstances sometimes take priority over your weight-management program, and write them down here (for example, "I want to keep food records, but I always eat on the run, so I never write things down"):

_____

_____

_____

_____

_____

Look at the list you just made, and write down some ways in which you can make your weight the priority over these factors (for example, "I need to make an agreement with myself that I will take 2 minutes each time I eat to determine portion sizes and calories, and to write down what I eat"):

_____

_____

_____

_____

_____

Good versus Evil
—Avoiding All-or-Nothing Thinking

George was a man who was unstoppable once he put his mind to something. This characteristic applied to projects at work, home repairs, and diet and physical activity programs. Once he got started, George got tunnel vision. He would work diligently and resist any temptation. When he was at his goal—and not a moment before—he would step back and admire the outcome. For many projects, this approach worked well. Some projects have a beginning and an end, and for those he could work unrelentingly until the end. At the end, he could relax.

With weight loss and weight maintenance, however, George had a problem. When he was "on," things went great. The pounds would melt off. When he "finished" his weight-loss project, though, George would inevitably relax. Almost immediately, the pounds would start piling back on, and soon he would be right back where he started. You see, George was either on a diet, or he was off it. For him, there was no in-between. Because weight maintenance is a lifelong process with no end, George never could keep the lost weight off.

Mandy, in contrast, would spend months trying to get up the momentum to start her diet and exercise program (she always started them at the same time; she couldn't start one without the other). When she finally got up the motivation to start, she would do a great job for a week or two. She felt great about the dry toast and baked fish, gallons of water, and hours of aerobics. But after a couple of weeks of near-neurotic perfection, she would start to think about the white chocolate chip chunks in the macadamia nut cookies. Her mouth would start to water and her stomach to growl. She could almost smell those cookies coming out of the oven, feel the soft-but-chewy cookie melting in her mouth, and taste the white chocolate as she licked it off her fingers. She would tremble inside at the thought. It was all so real.

And real it would become, for soon Mandy would buy the cookie, eat it, and thoroughly enjoy it. She would then be off to the races, guilt-ridden and eating every forbidden food around. The exercise clothes would soon be buried in the closet beneath her "fat clothes," as she called them. And she would end up 5 pounds heavier than when she started. For Mandy, this was a regular pattern.

One thing George and Mandy have in common is that they both suffer from all-or-nothing thinking. George sees weight loss as an on-or-off project. Mandy fails to see a situation for what it really is and suffers from perfectionistic thinking. Either she is great or she is awful. There is no in-between for either of them.

Each day we make many, many decisions regarding our weight (whether we are aware of them or not). For example, we choose what to eat at each meal, whether we will take the stairs or the elevator, whether or not to stop at the vending machines we pass twenty times a day, whether or not to go in any of the dozens of restaurants we pass, and whether we will buy a candy bar when we get gas. Do you see how many opportunities there are to stray from your eating and activity plans? With all this temptation, can you see why it is impossible to lose weight and keep it off with perfectionistic, all-or-nothing thinking?

The flip side is that there are also many, many opportunities in a day to make decisions in favor of weight management. Every time you pass a vending machine or restaurant without stopping, you have been a success. We don't often see this part of the weight-management picture. Because weight management is a lifelong process, you can expect that you will make both decisions that support weight management and those that do not. The favorable outcome occurs, though, when you make more good decisions than bad ones. The balance will show on the scale.

Although it is very difficult to change the way you think, it is also very important. You must become aware of the decisions you do make. If you are tempted by food in a vending machine, you must stop and recognize that you are making a decision either in favor of or against your weight-management plan. The decision to eat the food is a valid one, even if it pushes you over your calorie limit that day. You inevitably will make such choices at times. But when you do make those kinds of choices, it is important that you accept the decision as a valid one and move on. To stew on the decision and turn it into a statement about your inherent inability to lose weight is not valid. Further, it is not helpful to feel that because you were not perfect, you have the green light to eat any and all high-calorie foods.

What are some of the ways you exhibit all-or-nothing thinking?

_____

_____

_____

By completing this exercise, you have taken the first step in changing a thought pattern: to become aware of it. The next step is to challenge your thinking. For example, Mandy might recognize that she can follow a healthy, low-calorie diet to the letter. She also realizes that once she eats a single food item that she does not consider healthy and low-calorie, she goes on a binge. She thinks that she has failed and lost control. She starts to beat up on herself emotionally. In her head, she says things such as "Now you won't be able to get back to your diet. This day is a loss. You are so weak. You will never be able to stay on the diet. You may as well just write this day off and eat all the bad stuff you want."

Once she stops to recognize that she is having these thoughts, she should write down a rational (as opposed to emotional) response to her thoughts and behaviors. For example, she could state that what she did was a normal human response to delicious food. She is no different than most people just because she ate a white chocolate macadamia nut cookie. She also could calculate the actual number of calories she ate. She might find that she ate 250 calories in that cookie. If possible, she could deduct the calories elsewhere in the day. If not, she could simply realize that she ate 250 calories more than she wanted to that day, and realize that 250 calories is not enough to make or break a weight-loss program.

Another way for Mandy to look at this situation is to recognize that she will never have perfect eating and exercise habits. There will always be events that will interfere with her goals. The trick is to minimize the number of such events. Thanksgiving is a good example. On this holiday centered around eating, many people find it difficult to stick with their diets. However, Thanksgiving is only 1 day out of 365. What you do on the other 364 days is far more important than what you do on that 1 day.

Write down some rational thoughts in response to your all-or-nothing thinking in the above exercise:

_____

_____

_____

While you are in the process of learning new ways of thinking, practice this exercise for a 10-minute period each day. Reflect back on the day, and see where you engaged in all-or-nothing thinking.

Weight Loss Is Easy?
—Getting through the Maintenance Blahs

Most everyone knows that losing weight is a very difficult task. Anyone who has ever dieted can appreciate your efforts at weight loss. Many people are able to lose weight, however. And if statistics mean anything, weight loss is easy . . . compared with weight maintenance.

Weight loss is very difficult for many reasons. First, you are denying your body's basic drive to eat and meet certain calorie needs. You may be developing an entirely new way of coping with your feelings. You may have to learn new communication skills. All of these things require a lot of time and energy. For the weight-loss stage, though, there seems to be a beginning and an end—a finish line. For the maintenance stage, there is no end. It is a lifelong process.

Furthermore, while you are losing weight, you are getting rewarded by things like weight loss, new clothes, and compliments. During weight maintenance, this situation changes. You are working almost as hard *just to stay the same.* The compliments come less frequently. The clothes are no longer new. Perhaps some of the dreams that you thought would be realized when you got slim have not been fulfilled. This situation can be disheartening and can make the effort required to maintain your weight loss seem like torture at times.

At times you may ask yourself why you carry on. Is this really all it's cracked up to be? Part of the reason you are having these thoughts is because people tend to forget pain as they move away from it. Time heals wounds, including the wounds associated with being overweight. You must remember the reasons why you went through the weight-loss process to begin with.

You must remember how it felt when you could not find a chair to sit in; when the neighbor's child made fun of you; or when your doctor told you that if you didn't lose weight, you would have to take insulin. These are the reasons you started to lose weight in the first place.

You also may find it useful to think about—in fact, to write down—some of the advantages of being thin. Perhaps you can shop longer because your stamina has improved. Maybe you feel proud of your accomplishment. Perhaps your knee pain has abated. Have you started taking these things for granted? Have you forgotten that these things were not always a reality for you?

Next, it may be important to explore the reasons why maintaining your weight loss is so difficult for you at times. Are you still applying the skills you learned while you were trying to lose weight? Is maintaining a certain weight harder than you thought it would be? For example, did you realize that you would have to spend an hour a day, 5 days a week, exercising? Is this exercise regimen something that you really don't want to do? Are you living off of 1,700 calories a day to maintain this weight? Is this calorie level something you really don't want to maintain? Take these things into consideration. In the process of learning how to maintain your new, lower body weight, you may gain a few pounds. That may be okay. You will probably not follow all the diet principles perfectly. Remember that you are learning new skills and that you will stumble at times. The important thing is that you continue to practice new skills and to learn and grow based on this information.

Spend some time thinking about these questions:

What are the reasons you chose to lose weight? (For example, you may have wanted to have more confidence.)

_____

_____

_____

_____

What are the advantages of being at your current weight? (For example, you may be more able to keep up with your children.)

_____

_____

_____

_____

What are some of the disadvantages of being at your current weight? (For example, you have to count calories and don't get to eat some of your favorite foods.)

_____

_____

_____

_____

What are some ways to diminish the disadvantages? (For example, maybe you could save some calories so that you could include some of your favorite foods sometimes; or you could decide to eat 200 extra calories per day, knowing that you would gain ½ pound per week.)

_____

_____

_____

_____

Maintenance, which is the last—and longest—stage of the weight-loss journey, is conceivably the most important. Never think that the road will be without potholes. It has been said that there are some things people can learn only through tribulation, or that the only way out of a problem is to work through it. Too often in life people want to change, but they turn their backs on their desires when things get tough. They may delude themselves into thinking that they should postpone things—that somehow, it will be easier next time. So they hit the wall, turn back, hit the wall again, and turn back again. In weight control, the concept of *breakthrough* exists because it is only by persisting and gradually breaking through the wall that the dream of lifelong weight loss becomes a reality. It is hoped that this time you will decide that you will keep chipping at the wall, one choice at a time, until the dream becomes a reality.

APPENDIX A: WEEKLY PROGRESS SHEET

Name: _____

Goal weight: _____ Initial weight: _____

Date	Weight Change	Goal Met?	New Goals	Records Kept?	Days/Minutes of Physical Activity	Comments

APPENDIX B: GOAL RECORD SHEET

Write down your goal, and place a mark in the boxes for each day that you achieve that goal.

GOAL	Mon.	Tues.	Wed.	Thurs.	Fri.	Sat.	Sun.	Mon.	Tues.	Wed.	Thurs.	Fri.	Sat.	Sun.
Eat a lunch of less than 300 calories	✔	✔	✔	✔	✔			✔	✔	✔	✔	✔		
Walk 30 minutes		✔	✔	✔		✔	✔	✔	✔		✔	✔		
Eat baby carrots for a snack		✔	✔	✔					✔	✔				
Keep snack cakes out of the house	✔	✔	✔	✔	✔	✔	✔	✔	✔	✔	✔	✔	✔	✔

GOAL RECORD SHEET

Write down your goal, and place a mark in the boxes for each day that you achieve that goal.

GOAL	Mon.	Tues.	Wed.	Thurs.	Fri.	Sat.	Sun.	Mon.	Tues.	Wed.	Thurs.	Fri.	Sat.	Sun.

APPENDIX C: FOOD RECORD

Name: _____

Date: _____

Time	Food and Portion Size	Calories	Hunger*	Mood	With	Where	Running Daily Calorie Total

*Scale of 1 to 5, with 5 being the most hungry.

Total daily calories: _____   Calories burned in physical activity (calculate using Table 2) : _____

Physical activity: _____   Weekly weight: _____